A JEWISH PHYSICIAN'S RESPONSE TO THE BLACK DEATH

FOUNDATIONS

Further Information and Publications

www.arc-humanities.org/series/book-series/

A JEWISH PHYSICIAN'S RESPONSE TO THE BLACK DEATH

ABRAHAM CASLARI'S *TRACTATE ON PESTILENTIAL FEVERS AND FEVER TYPES*

Edited and translated by

SUSAN L. EINBINDER

ARC HUMANITIES PRESS

British Library Cataloguing in Publication Data
A catalogue record for this book is available from the British Library.

ISBN (Hardback): 9781802703979
e-ISBN (PDF): 9781802704730
e-ISBN (EPUB): 9781802704747

DOI: 10.17302/dohf2085

www.arc-humanities.org

Printed and bound in the UK (by CPIGroup [UK] Ltd), USA (by Bookmasters), and elsewhere using print-on-demand technology.

Publisher (manufacturer) details: Arc Humanities Press, 14 Clifton Moor Business Village, James Nicolson Link, York YO30 4XG, United Kingdom.

EU Authorized Representative details (for GPSR purposes): Amsterdam University Press, Nieuwe Prinsengracht 89, 1018 VR Amsterdam, The Netherlands. www.aup.nl

CONTENTS

THE TEXTS: TRANSCRIPTIONS AND TRANSLATIONS

DOI: 10.17302/dohf20851 © Arc Humanities Press, 2026

LIST OF ILLUSTRATIONS

DOI: 10.17302/dohf20852 © Arc Humanities Press, 2026

PREFACE

> I saw that if I did not make clearly known these fevers—what type they are—the truth of my opinion about their treatment would not be disseminated.
>
> Abraham b. David Caslari
> *Tractate on Pestilential Fevers and Fever Types*

I NEVER INTENDED to produce a critical edition of a medieval medical treatise. The author of the treatise in question, Abraham b. David Caslari, began his professional career as a young man in or near Narbonne, where his father was also a physician and admirer of the local literary figures writing in Hebrew in the early fourteenth century. Philip IV's royal decree of expulsion sent Abraham, his wife, father, and approximately 100,000 French Jews into exile. Most of those exiles, especially from northern France, disappeared without a trace. In contrast, with the advantages of location, a welcoming reception from the kingdom of Aragon, professional skills in demand, and a notable degree of personal ambition, Abraham remains visible in the documentary record over the next four decades. We can follow him from Provence to Perpignan into Catalonia, where after several years he landed in Besalú, not far from Girona. He disappears in 1349, perhaps, as I argue, a victim of the Black Death. Before the plague silenced him, however, he had treated some of its victims and was confident that he was curing them. My first encounter with Abraham was through the composition that makes this claim, his third and final extant medical work, the *Tractate on Pestilential Fevers and Fever Types*; Abraham and a discussion of his tractate merited a chapter in my book, *After the Black Death*. Long after that book's publication in 2018, however, I remained dissatisfied with the limitations of that treatment; I was convinced that there was more to say about Abraham, his theories, and his experience during the Black Death.

Thus, my initial intention was to write more *about* Abraham b. David Caslari. Nonetheless, that would have compelled readers to rely on my say-so about the contents of his tractate, which was central to the reconstruction I envisioned. That seemed unfair, as did the inexplicable unavailability of this remarkable work to modern readers: hence a detour to this book.

DOI: 10.17302/dohf20853

I am acutely aware that I am not a trained text editor, a paleographer, philologist, or codicologist, and some of you will find fault with my failure to treat those features of the manuscript copies more fully. What is lacking I deeply hope that others will come along to provide. I have, however, leaned heavily on the skills I have developed over decades of work as a literary scholar, historian, and, more recently, as one of a cohort of scholars rewriting the story of plague and of the Black Death.

This work will surely find emendation over time, maybe even by me. What matters is that Abraham himself, in Hebrew and in my English translations, is now able to do what he fervently wished: to disseminate his views to generations to come. As he also said, his readers were free to agree or disagree with him, but they should share his belief that the "signs" led to the truth. His openness to dissent, and his faith in the facts, are enviable today.

ACKNOWLEDGEMENTS

TO WRITE A scholarly book is invariably to amass debts to libraries, librarians, and generous colleagues. Among the libraries, I am grateful to the University of Connecticut's Homer Babbidge Library; to Brown University's Rockefeller Library; and to the National Library of Israel in Jerusalem, especially to its Institute for Microfilmed Hebrew Manuscripts and KTIV database of digitized Hebrew manuscripts from around the world. Among librarians, I owe special thanks to Michael Young and Joe Natale at UConn and to Yael Okun and Alexander Gordin at the IMHM and NLI, respectively. Among the colleagues whose patience and generosity were indefatigable, I owe thanks to Gerrit Bos, Ann Carmichael, Lola Ferre, Nahyan Fancy, Monica H. Green, Michael McVaugh, Anne van Arsdall, and Yossi (Joseph) Ziegler. Lola was greatly helpful going over rough spots in my translations, as was Michael as a sounding board. Also invaluable were those colleagues who were not historians of medicine but listeners, critics, and cheerleaders: Carolyn Betensky, Caroline W. Bynum, Alan Cooper, Margot Fassler, Tyler Franconi, Susan Harvey, and Sallie Spence. Thank you also to Danna Messer, Tania Colwell, and Martine Maguire-Weltecke at Arc Humanities Press for their willingness to take on this project and for their guidance; and to Christina Dedora, Cheryl Pynn-Dedora, and Kathy Taylor of Sanctuary Herbs in Cranston, RI, for teaching me about herbs and healing.

Thank you to Brown University's Department of Religious Studies, which has kindly afforded me visiting scholar status for several years. Early forays into aspects of Abraham's tractate were presented at the American Association for Historians of Medicine (Kansas City, 2024) and the Medieval Academy of America (Cambridge, MA, 2025). Thank you to both organizations for providing a forum for my work.

Finally, Abraham b. David Caslari's insistence that I still had more to do with him has kept him close for almost a decade, and I am grateful, too, to this remarkable if neglected medieval Jewish physician. The importance of bringing Abraham into the conversation of scholars who could not access him in Hebrew overrode my hesitation to be his intermediary. His story is in some respect all of ours: at a time when scholars, scientists and physicians, refugees and immigrants are increasingly under threat, I note that Abraham

DOI: 10.17302/dohf20854 © Arc Humanities Press, 2026

belonged to every one of these categories. Hopefully, this book will introduce him to new admirers and friends.

In true acknowledgement form, I will close by saying whatever help and inspiration have made this work possible, its errors are mine alone: I also acknowledge my debt to those of you who will come along later and improve what I have done. Abraham b. David Caslari, who so feared being consigned to oblivion, awaits you.

Providence, RI. December 19, 2025.

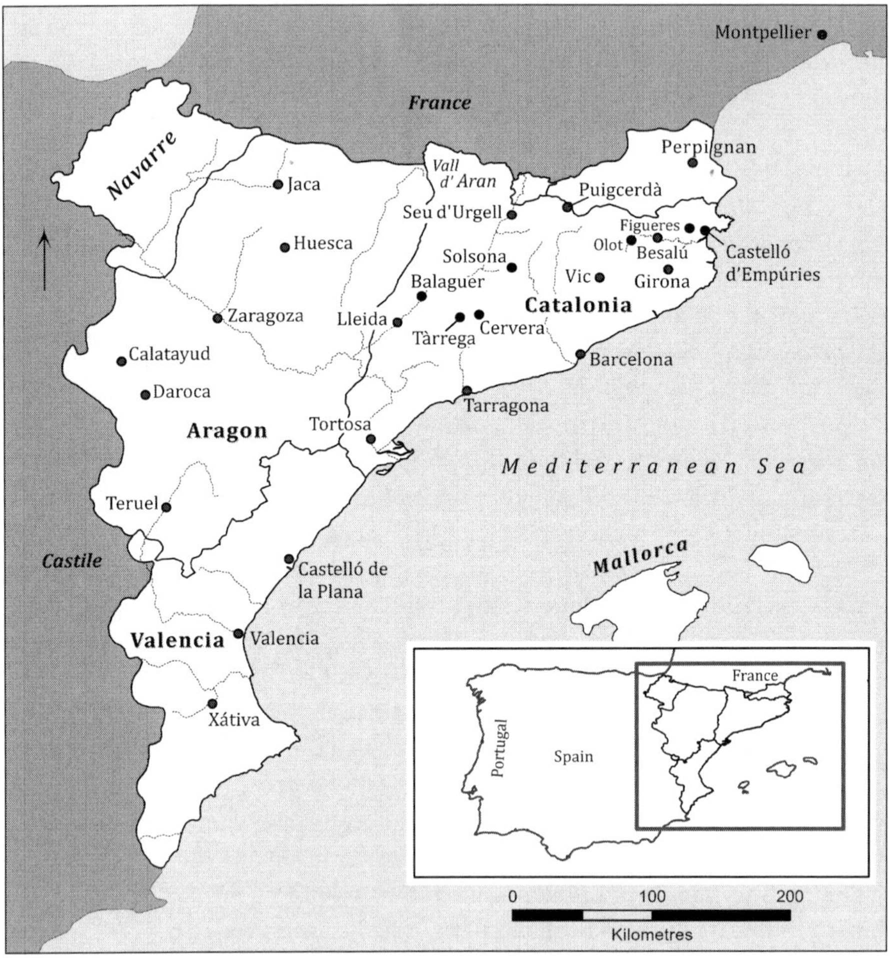

Figure 1. A map of the Crown of Aragon and Catalonia, ca. 1300. Map by Gordon Thompson, 2025. Reproduced with permission.

ABRAHAM CASLARI'S *TRACTATE ON PESTILENTIAL FEVERS AND FEVER TYPES*

LOOKING BACK ON the past year, Abraham Caslari might have summoned one consolation: most of *his* patients had lived. Although his colleagues had not been so fortunate, they still rejected his diagnosis of the recent fevers and his approach to treating them. Abraham's defiant response was directed primarily to them, but it has bequeathed us one of the earliest responses to the Black Death by a contemporary physician. Long noted but undertreated, in this study Abraham's *Tractate on Pestilential Fevers and Fever Types* finds its first critical edition, English translation, and serious treatment.[1]

As it has come down to us, Abraham's tractate raises many questions, beginning with his rejection of an emerging consensus that the fevers of 1348–1349 were pestilential. Was Abraham's repudiation of that diagnosis theoretical or rooted in experience, and why did he insist that bleeding and purging plague victims were critical to their cure? Who were the contemporary readers Abraham sought to address and what did later readers make of his argument? What, if any, impact did Abraham and Jewish physicians like him have in the contentious debates over the identity of the Black Death fevers? For modern readers, the most common association of Jews and the Black Death is the sweeping violence against Jewish communities that accompanied the plague across Aragon and Catalonia. Indeed, that violence embeds Abraham's text in a traumatic moment in Jewish history—but does it echo in Abraham's work? The following essay touches upon these and other questions, providing for the first time a full transcription and annotated translation of the *Tractate*. Although the work's existence has been noted for many years, references to it in secondary sources, including occasional citations, have been dependent either on a faulty 1891 edition by Herman Pinkhof or recycled from excerpts or opinions found in other studies.[2]

---

1 The Hebrew title, which appears only on one of the two extant copies, is מאמר על קדחות דבריות ומיני הקדחות. The two extant sources are Paris, Bibliothèque nationale de France (hereafter BnF), MS héb. 1191, fols. 115a–123b (NLI, IMHM F 14747) and Leiden, Leiden University Library, MS or. 4778, fols. 134b–141a (NLI, IMHM F 17378).

2 Jon Arrizabalaga, "Facing the Black Death: Perceptions and Reactions of University

DOI: 10.17302/dohf20855 © Arc Humanities Press, 2026

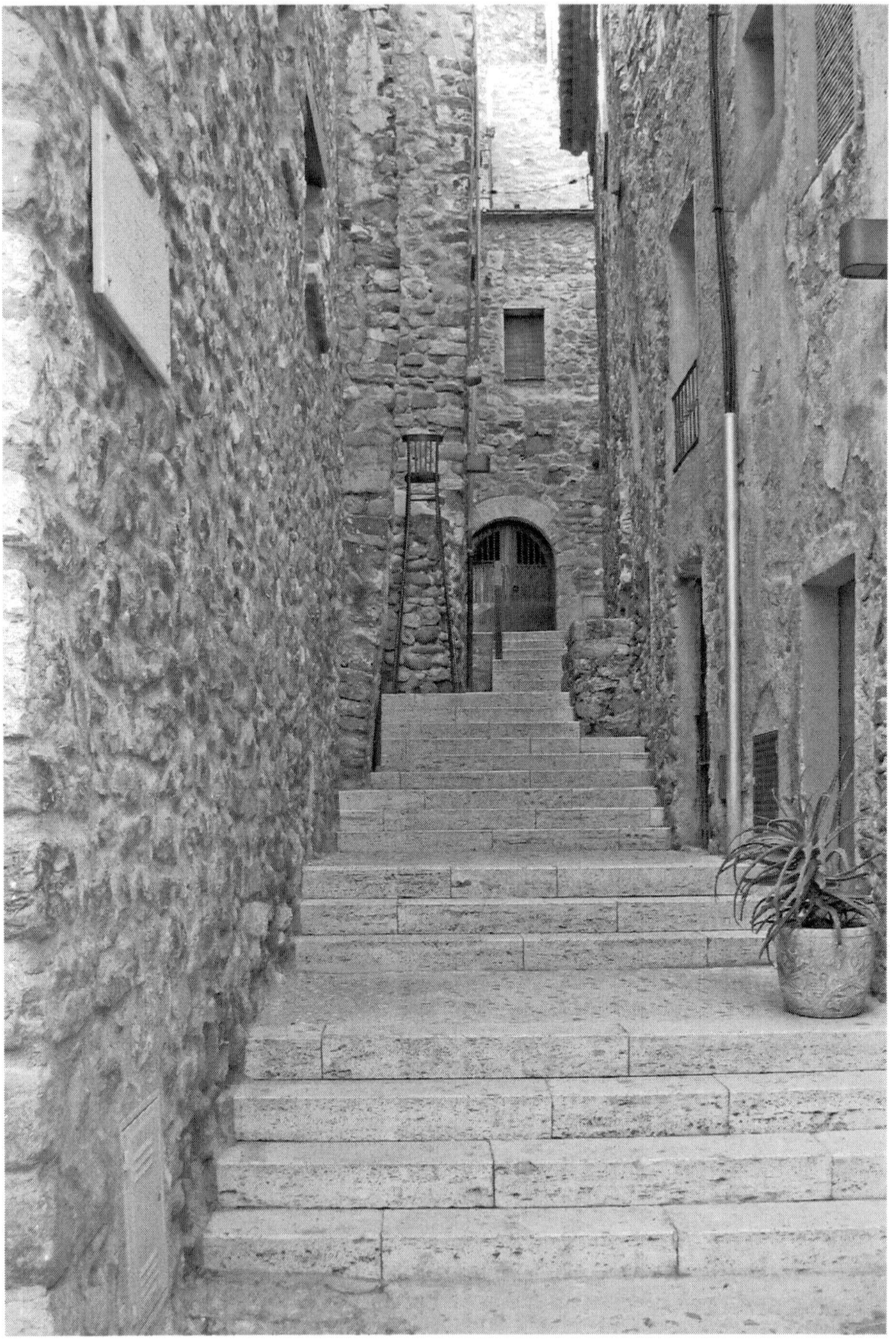

Figure 2. "Abraham Caslari Street" in the medieval Jewish *call*, or quarter, of Besalú. Image courtesy of Creative Commons and through the GNU Free Documentation License. Photograph by Naevus. CC BY-SA 3.0.

A recent book by John Aberth, aimed at a general audience, recognizes the tractate's significance but misrepresents most of what Abraham Caslari wrote.[3] For years, rumours circulated that a critical edition was underway, but they have not been realized.[4] Direct access to the text is overdue and this edition hopefully will make it accessible to scholars and lay readers interested in the medical, historical, environmental, and cultural dimensions of premodern plague. The threads I am unable or have chosen not to pursue are theirs to follow.

The Black Death in Catalonia

The fevers that Abraham Caslari confronted from the spring of 1348 into the next summer were lethal and moved swiftly. Both their lethality and speed are still not fully understood, and until recently were regularly invoked by a handful of historians skeptical that the Black Death was caused by bubonic plague. One of the remarkable milestones of plague scholarship, however, has been the genetic sequencing of ancient DNA (aDNA) in human remains from the graves of plague victims.[5] Preserved for centuries in dental pulp, aDNA proved that *Yersinia pestis*, the plague bacillus, was the pathogen behind the three major pandemics of historical record: the First (Justinianic) Pandemic spanning the mid-sixth to eighth centuries; the Second (Black Death) Pandemic spanning the mid-fourteenth to mid-eighteenth centuries; and the Third Pandemic spanning from the late nineteenth century to the

Medical Practitioners," in Luis García Ballester et al., eds., *Practical Medicine from Salerno to the Black Death* (Cambridge: Cambridge University Press, 1994), 237–88; Ron Barkai, "Jewish Treatises on the Black Death, 1300–1500: A Preliminary Study," in Roger French et al., eds., *Medicine from the Black Death to the French Disease* (Aldershot: Ashgate, 1998), 6–25; Susan L. Einbinder, *After the Black Death: Plague and Commemoration among Iberian Jews* (Philadelphia: University of Pennsylvania Press, 2018); H. Pinkhof, *Abraham Kashlari over pestachtige koortsen. Hebreeuwsch met Nederlandsche vertaling. Naar het te Leidenvoorhanden handschrift, benevens een bericht over vier andere 14e eeuwsche Hebreeuwsche handschriften, handelende overde pest* (Amsterdam, 1891).

3 John Aberth, *Doctoring the Black Death: Medieval Europe's Medical Response to Plague* (Lanham: Rowman & Littlefield, 2021).

4 In 2011, Gerrit Bos and Guido Mensching referred to a forthcoming edition in preparation by Jessica Kley. Gerrit Bos and Guido Mensching, "The Black Death in Hebrew Literature: Abraham Ben Solomon Hen's *Tractatulus de Pestilentia*," *Jewish Studies Quarterly* 18 (2011): 34n10.

5 Kirsten I. Bos et al., "A Draft Genome of *Yersinia pestis* from Victims of the Black Death," *Nature* 478 (2011): 506–10.

present day.[6] Genomic sequencing also offered a way to track the evolving adaptation of *Y. pestis* to new hosts and ecosystems as it journeyed across continents and species. This ongoing work constantly revises what we know about plague in general and the Second Pandemic—heralded spectacularly by the Black Death—in particular.

As the example of Abraham Caslari shows, rewriting Black Death history extends also to the role of Jewish physicians in their medical and social contexts. *The Tractate on Pestilential Fevers and Fever Types* attests to the existence of a Jewish textual community, writing in Hebrew and shaped by the interests, language, and norms of scholastic university medicine. The anti-Jewish violence of 1348–1349 may have frayed the ties between Jewish and Christian medical practitioners, but in Abraham's case, at least, it does not seem to have frayed his allegiance to what they taught or his desire to emulate them.

According to the received historical narrative, the Black Death "began" somewhere in "the east," making its way to Crimea and the Black Sea by the mid-1340s. Recent paleogenetic studies have identified the Tian Shan mountains, near what is now Kyrgyzstan, as the likely origin for a spillover from marmot populations to Mongol traders or invaders, although possibly much earlier than the 1330s dates preserved on gravestones in the area.[7] The old story had plague move with the Mongols to the port of Caffa, where it infected Genoese merchants under siege. The Genoese merchants fled to

---

6 In fact, aDNA sequencing has identified plague in LNBA (Late Neolithic Bronze Age) remains, also, documenting a strain of *Y. pestis* that had not yet developed the ability to enlist an intermediate arthropod vector (flea, lice, tick) en route to a mammal host. See, for example, Aida Andrades Valtueña et al., "The Stone Age Plague and its Persistence in Eurasia," *Current Biology* 27 (2017): 3683–89; Simon Rasmussen et al., "Early Divergent Strains of *Yersinia Pestis* in Eurasia 5000 Years Ago," *Cell* 153 (2015): 571–82; Daniel Weiss, "Bronze Age Plague," *Archaeology* Jan/Feb 2019, https://archaeology.org/issues/january-february-2019/collection/russia-samara-bronze-age-plague/top-10-discoveries-of-2018/. On Second Pandemic chronology, as noted below, the Second Pandemic may have reached the Middle East earlier, by the mid-thirteenth century, and entered Europe early in the fourteenth century. See Nahyan Fancy and Monica H. Green, "Plague and the Fall of Baghdad (1258)," *Medical History* 65, no. 2 (2021): 155–77.

7 Maria A. Spyrou et al., "The Source of the Black Death in Fourteenth-Century Central Eurasia," *Nature* 606 (2022): 718–24; Marcel Keller et al., "A Refined Phylochronology of the Second Plague Pandemic in Western Eurasia," preprint *bioRxv*, July 19, 2023, doi.org/10.1101/2023.07.18.549544; Monica H. Green, "Out of the East (or North or South): A Response to Philip Slavin," *Past & Present* 256, no. 1 (2022): 283–323; Monica Green and Andre Oliveira da Silva, "Shifting Paradigms in Black Death Chronologies," *Hypotheses*, May 23, 2023, https://urbrel.hypotheses.org/5550.

Sicily, then Marseille, carrying plague, which then began its historic sweep across Europe. As Hannah Barker has shown, the transmission of plague to Europe in 1347 probably owed more to the lifting of grain embargoes in Tana, on the other side of the Azov Sea, than to the siege of Caffa.[8] Historian Monica H. Green has argued persuasively that plague was likely on the move decades before the 1340s, and from different directions. How to interpret the genetic evidence, and how to integrate it with more traditional historical sources, are more contentious questions.

What is certain, however, is that what happened in Europe between 1347–1353 unfolded with a speed and ferocity unmatched by previous or successive outbreaks. Mortality estimates for Europe, where most research has focused, range from 30–90 or even 100% depending on the locale. For the Middle East, chroniclers, religious leaders, and physicians describe staggering mortality, and if their numbers cannot always be taken literally, other written and material sources support the case for devastating losses; for Africa and Asia, where sources are scarcer, collateral evidence implies high mortality also.[9] The older studies of plague's impact in Iberia produced contradictory assessments, generalizing about variable mortality in the mountains (low mortality) versus the plains (high), the cities (high) versus the villages (low). Several important studies looked at the high mortality rates among different professional groups—notaries in Perpignan, for instance, or clerics in Barcelona.[10] Indisputably, many professional men in what we

8 Hannah Barker, "Laying the Corpses to Rest: Grain, Embargoes, and *Yersinia pestis* in the Black Sea, 1346–1348," *Speculum* 96, no. 1 (2021): 97–126.

9 Gerard Chouin, "Reflections on Plague in African History (14th–19th century)," *Afriques* 9 (2018), https://doi.org/10.4000/afriques.2228; Michael Dols, *The Black Death in the Midde East* (Princeton: Princeton University Press, 1977); Monica H. Green, "Four Black Deaths," *American Historical Review* 125, no. 5 (2020): 1601–31; Green, "Putting Africa on the Black Death Map: Narratives from Genetics and History," *Afriques* 9 (2018), https://doi.org/10.4000/afriques.2125; Green and Oliveira da Silva, "Shifting Paradigms"; Robert Hymes and Monica H. Green, *New Evidence for the Dating and Impact of the Black Death in Asia*, ed. Carol Symes, *The Medieval Globe* (Arc Humanities, 2022).

10 Jaume Sobreques Callico, "La pesta negra en la peninsula Iberica," *Anuario de estudios medievales* 7 (1970–1971): 67–102; Richard Emery, "The Black Death in Perpignan," *Speculum* 42 no. 4 (1967): 611–23; Richard Gyug, "The Effects and Extent of the Black Death of 1348: New Evidence for Clerical Mortality in Barcelona," *Mediaeval Studies* 45, no. 1 (1983): 385–96; William D. Phillips, "Peste negra: The Fourteenth-Century Plague Epidemics in Iberia," in *On the Social Origins of Medieval Institutions*, eds. Donald Kagay and T. M. Vann (Leiden: Brill, 1998), 47–62. For archaeological evidence, see Julie Beltrán de Heredia Bercero and I. Gibrat Pineda,

call frontline work tried to keep doing their jobs. Physicians died, too, like Jacme d'Agramont in Lleida, whose Catalan tractate detailed prophylactic measures to the councillors of that city.[11] Many other physicians, surgeons, barbers, and lay healers whose names have been lost, gave their lives tending to the sick. Municipalities in Aragon were already contracting with physicians to treat their residents before the Black Death; as early as 1315, Abraham Caslari served in this capacity in Castelló d'Empúries, an autonomous territory neighbouring Besalú.[12] His plague tractate testifies that he had treated plague patients during the Black Death, presumably there and in Besalú.

Physicians, clerics, and notaries were not the plague's only first responders. Boccaccio's account of the dissolution of family and social ties among plague-terrorized communities had a lasting impact both as a literary topos and as a description of social reality unquestioned by later readers. In a groundbreaking study the historian Shona Wray argued that family members desperately tried to care for parents, children, and neighbours; communities also struggled valiantly to bury the dead with a modicum of dignity, sometimes to bury them at all. When the wave of deaths tapered in the early 1350s, there were shortages of notaries, healers, teachers, farmers, clerics, and artisans. Orphans abounded, either destitute or with inheritances that less scrupulous souls were eager to oversee.[13] Elsewhere, people prayed their way through the pandemic and sometimes out the other side; they

---

"El primer testimoni arqueològic de la Pesta negra a Barcelona: La fossa comuna de la basília dels Sants Màrtirs Just i Pastor," *Quarhis* 2 no. 10 (2014): 164–75; Sacha Kacki and Dominique Castex, "La sépulture multiple de la basilique des saints martyrs Just et Pastor: Bio-archéologie des restes humaines," *Quarhis: Quaderns d'arqueologia i història de la ciutat de Barcelona* 2, no. 10 (2014): 180–99.

11 Arrizabalaga, "Facing the Black Death"; Joan Veny i Clar and F. Cremades, eds., *Regiment de preservació de pestilència (1348): Jacme d'Agramont (nova edició)* (Barcelona: Universitat de Barcelona, 2015); C. E. Winslow and M. L. Duran-Reynals, "Jacme d'Agramont and the First of the Plague Tractates," *Bulletin of the History of Medicine* 22 (1948): 747–65.

12 According to Michael McVaugh, 1316: "El món medic de Castelló d'Empúries a principis del segle XIV," *Mot se razo* 10–11 (2012): 13.

13 Daniel Lord Smail has described the moving plight of Alayseta, a young woman in Marseille who appealed for leniency after failing to file as the sole heir to her father's estate. Alayseta had been too overwhelmed to collect the paperwork and make the journey to court, and a compassionate judge granted her an extension. Daniel Lord Smail, "A Life in the Black Death: The Inventory of Alayseta Paula (Marseille 1348)," https://middleagesforeducators.princeton.edu/life-black-death-inventory-alayseta-paula-marseille-1348.

supplemented their prayers with amulets, icons, relics, and processions, immune-boosting diets, and charitable bequests.

Historians have posited plague taking two paths through the Iberian Peninsula, one via the Pyrenees into Barcelona then moving west and northward, and one from Mallorca into Almeria heading south and west.[14] The textual sources have been supplemented by the excavations of several mass burials where aDNA has conclusively confirmed the presence of *Yersinia pestis* in human remains. One site, Just y Pastor outside Barcelona, has yielded an early Second Pandemic genome from remains carbon-dated to bracket a fourteenth-century event.[15] A mass grave in Tàrrega, about seventy miles (112.65 kilometres) west of Barcelona, unearthed 50-some individuals subsequently identified as Jewish victims of plague-inspired violence in 1348.

The theme of anti-Jewish violence recurs in all historical accounts of the Black Death and has dwarfed other dimensions of Jewish plague experience including that of their physicians. As noted above, the Black Death reached Barcelona in the spring of 1348, probably preceded by rumours implicating the Jews in its spread. On May 17, the Barcelona Jewish *call*, or quarter, was violently attacked, properties were plundered and destroyed, nineteen Jews were killed and an unrecorded number of victims wounded. The violence rippled westward, even as King Pere III ordered municipal authorities to protect local Jews (who were legally the property of the Crown and due royal protection) and punish malefactors. Local compliance varied. In Cervera, authorities protected their Jews; other towns, including Lleida, failed to do so. The worst episode occurred in Tàrrega, about seventy miles (ca. 113 kilometres) west of Barcelona, where the call was attacked in early July, according to a surviving chronicle account leaving three hundred dead.[16]

14 Andre Oliveira da Silva, "Chronologies, Routes and Conditions for the Spread of Plague in Portugal during the Black Death," *Anais de história de Além-Mar* 22 (2021): 59–84.

15 Shona Wray, "Tracking Family and Flight in Bologna during the Black Death," *Medieval People* 25, no. 1 (2004), article 7, https://scholarworks.wmich.edu/medpros/vol25/iss1/7; Wray, "Boccaccio and the Doctors: Medicine and Compassion in the Face of Plague," *Journal of Medieval History* 30, no. 3 (2004): 301–22; Wray, *Communities and Crisis: Bologna during the Black Death* (Leiden: Brill, 2009); Beltrán and Pineda, "El primer testimoni arqueològic"; Kacki and Castex, "La sépulture multiple"; Anna Colet et al., "The Black Death and its Consequences for the Jewish Community in Tàrrega: Lessons from History and Archeology," in Monica H. Green, ed., *Pandemic Disease in the Medieval World* special issue, *The Medieval Globe* 1 (2014): 63–96; Einbinder, *After the Black Death.*

16 I draw on my account in *After the Black Death*, ch. 5, especially 117–22. For painstaking reconstruction of events preceding and following the violence in

A long, weary period followed marked by petitions from survivors who had successfully fled to other towns, half-hearted prosecutions of perpetrators, attempts to retrieve auctioned Jewish goods and property, and royal enticements to the scattered survivors and newcomers to rebuild the *aljama*.

Recent studies by Tzafrir Barzilay and Monica H. Green have convincingly argued that the attacks should be linked to the violence against Jews and lepers some twenty years earlier, during the so-called Lepers Plot of 1321; Green's claims for "prodromic" outbreaks of plague prior to 1348 constitute a piece of this argument. The cause of the violence, which also characterized the Black Death's movement across central Europe and particularly what are now Germany and Austria, is not our topic here. Rather, what matters for this introduction is that violence against Jewish communities, causing loss of life and property, the displacement of survivors and the activation of Jewish networks of communication, advocacy, and undoubtedly relief, crisscrossed the cities, villages, and towns around Girona (which also experienced anti-Jewish violence) and Besalú.

In other words, Abraham Caslari in Besalú must have known about the cascading attacks on Catalonian Jewish communities, including Barcelona and Girona, and was treating patients in the shadow of that knowledge. The *Tractate on Pestilential Fevers and Fever Types* never alludes directly to social unrest, violence, or sectarian tensions. Nonetheless, Abraham's Hebrew description of the pandemic's movement echoes Hayim Galipapa's contemporary or near-contemporary chronicle of anti-Jewish attacks.[17] Whether that echo was consciously invoked to remind Hebrew readers that sickness rippled across Catalonia and Aragon accompanied by lethal violence is a good question. The answer depends on how we understand Abraham Caslari, and one way to try to do that is to read what he wrote. A medical tractate is not as yielding in this pursuit as a chronicle, testament, or verse, but like all these genres, it balances genre conventions against more idiosyncratic and personal impulses and perspectives. Even a medical tractate,

---

Tàrrega, see the studies by Josep Xavier Muntané listed in the bibliography. Since the entire *aljama* counted several hundred Jews, the tally may have included Jews from neighbouring villages as well. The mass graves discovered twenty years ago were only partially excavated, in part due to physical limitations accessing the terrain, and in part due to opposition from European Jewish rabbinic and regional authorities opposed to the disinterment of the bodies.

17 Einbinder, *After the Black Death*; Tzafrir Barzilay, "The Black Death in Aragon: Notes on a Jewish Chronicle" [in Hebrew], *Hayo Haya* 8 (2011): 53–71.

in other words, does not entirely efface its author, and in Abraham's case, we find an author who had no desire to be effaced.

The crux of Abraham's medical argument is his conviction that the fevers of 1348 were not what the received literature defined as "pestilence" but humoral in origin. Pestilential fevers were uniquely generated by a poisonous corruption or putrefaction of the air.[18] Humoral fevers, in contrast, were generated by a humoral imbalance that caused an excess of humour that in turn generated excess heat. Abraham blamed the humoral imbalance, or dyscrasia, that generated the 1348 fevers on subsistence shortages triggered by poor harvests and high prices that caused widespread malnutrition—a glimpse of environmental and social stresses that may have additionally contributed to intercommunal tensions. Abraham emphasized that while famine-induced fevers might be transmissible (what we call "contagious"), the altered quality of the air that could produce them was not inherently pestilential; the same, he argues, was even true of planetary conjunctions conventionally associated with pestilence. In all cases, God ultimately decided to make conditions pestilential or not.[19] As for the putrefaction in the humours that generated the recent fevers, Abraham claims that it was irrelevant whether putrefaction originated in a humour, spilled over to the blood and was then carried to the heart, or whether it originated in the heart and spilled over from the blood to the adjacent member and its associated humour. The extra toxicity of the fever gave it its pestilential qualities and explained some of the signs and symptoms that resembled those of true (i.e., unadulterated) pestilence. All this may seem today like pointless hairsplitting, but determining causation was the first step to understanding a patient's prognosis and treatment options.[20] Abraham's corollary argument was his insistence that bloodletting (phlebotomy), traditionally advised for humoral fevers but not for pestilential ones, was obligatory for treating the recent fevers.

18 Caslari uses the Hebrew word *dever* for pestilence. The biblical term referred to an unspecified but collectively experienced disease event inflicted by God as chastisement. With the Black Death, it would become specifically associated with bubonic plague.

19 Leiden, MS or. 4778, fol. 118a, with the corresponding passage in Paris, MS héb. 1191, fol. 138a.

20 According to Demaitre, the famous Montpellier faculty physician, Bernard de Gordon, especially emphasized the importance of knowing the cause of a disease to treat it. Luke Demaitre, *Doctor Bernard de Gordon, Professor and Practitioner* (Toronto: Pontifical Institute of Mediaeval Studies, 1980), 132.

What Abraham saw in his and his colleagues' patients, therefore, shaped his medical argument as much as his learning did: his tractate is not merely a theoretical exercise but an attempt to reconcile theoretical models with real-life experience. Whether or not bubonic plague was new to Catalonia in 1348, it was new on the horrific scale of that year. The social and environmental factors that Abraham thought relevant to its emergence and behaviour, and the form and language he enlisted to prove his case, make his treatise a document of social and literary, as well as medical, history. Like his seeming silence on the violence against Jewish communities, Abraham's stubborn repudiation of the medical consensus taking shape among his peers adds intrigue to his story. A lifetime of thinking and experience lie behind *The Tractate on Pestilential Fevers and Fever Types*, illuminating an early and learned attempt to grapple with the Black Death and by extension some of the turbulent context that gave it birth.

Despite its technical language, the *Tractate* is also, and self-consciously, a literary construct, meaning not that it is fiction but that it could not be written without attention to conventions of language, format, affect, and style. In this context, the *Tractate*'s display of authority, erudition, and occasional indignation are part of its design; they illuminate an authorial persona that reveals glimpses of the private man and the private, public, and professional worlds he sought to navigate in a time of crisis. What he included or omitted, and what his sense of genre permitted him to include or omit, created an image of its author as well as *The Tractate on Pestilential Fevers and Fever Types*.

Abraham b. David Caslari

What we know about Abraham Caslari's personal life is patchy but not insignificant. The royal decree that sent 100,000 to 150,000 French Jews in panic-stricken flight from homes they had known for generations included the Jews of Narbonne in Languedoc, where Abraham, his father David, and their families lived.[21] Henri Gross thought that the family name, Caslari, referred to the village of Castlar not far from Narbonne, and it may be that this Caslari family originated there.[22] David Caslari, Abraham's father, was a physician in

---

21 William C. Jordan, *The French Monarchy and the Jews* (Philadelphia: University of Pennsylvania Press, 1989); Jordan, "Administering Expulsion in 1306," *Jewish Studies Quarterly* 15, no. 3 (2008): 241–50.

22 Henri Gross, *Gallia Judaica* (Paris: Cerf, 1897), 618–21. Other Caslaris, contemporary but unrelated, like Israel b. Joseph Caslari and Crescas Caslari, came

Narbonne intimately connected to the local intellectual and literary Jewish elite. He was praised by the local poet and rhetorician, Abraham Bedersi, who enlisted him to judge a poetic competition. Closer to his professional expertise, he also produced a Hebrew translation of a Latin version of Galen's *Peri Anomalou Dyskrasias*, a short treatise on humoral imbalance that is extant today.[23] The father's interests benefited from his location in a hub of medical learning and activity centred in nearby Montpellier. Similarly, his connections to Narbonne's Jewish literary elite testify to broader interests including an appreciation for belletristic Hebrew—although the extravagant formalism esteemed by Bedersi and his circle locates contemporary aesthetic appeal far from our own. Ironically, the Hebrew of David's translation is at times incomprehensible:[24] Like many fellow Jewish physicians who tried their hand at translating the medical texts at the core of the Christian university curriculum, he struggled to express in Hebrew the scientific and philosophical concepts that language had not yet evolved to convey. Clearly, David knew some Latin, and apparently Abraham did as well. Indeed, Abraham was probably tutored by his father, as Jews were not permitted to attend the universities. Most Jewish physicians taught and trained their sons, combining clinical supervision with readings translated from the core university curriculum.[25] David and Abraham Caslari, talented, intellectually inclined, and professionally ambitious, followed the curricular trends at Montpellier avidly.

Many, if not most, French Jews disappeared without a trace in the wake of the Great Expulsion of 1306. Thousands converted, and those who fled were simply too far from the borders of possible harbour. Most of the Jews of Narbonne crowded into nearby Perpignan, at the time under Aragonese rule, and from there fanned out into Aragon and Catalonia. David, Abraham, and their families initially made their way from Perpignan to Lleida, relocating a few years later to Besalú. David died in 1315, but Abraham steadily

from Narbonne or nearby; they were authors and translators in their own right. See Susan L. Einbinder, *No Place of Rest: Jewish Literature, Expulsion, and the Memory of Medieval France* (Philadelphia: University of Pennsylvania Press, 2008).

23 Gerrit Bos et al., *Transmitting a Text through Three Languages: The Future History of Galen's Peri Anomalou Dyskrasias* (Philadelphia: Transactions of the American Philosophical Society, 2014), n.s., 104, no. 5: 1–168.

24 Bos et al., *Transmitting a Text through Three Languages*.

25 Alternatively, parents might contract with a Jewish physician to teach and apprentice their son. Joseph Shatzmiller, "Apprenticeship or Academic Education: The Making of Jewish Doctors," in *Schüler und Meister*, eds. Andreas Speer and Thomas Jeschke (Berlin: De Gruyter, 2016), 503–10; Einbinder, *After the Black Death*, 67.

amassed wealth and a professional reputation that have left multiple traces in royal and local archives. In 1320, he requested and received royal permission to marry a second wife (while still married to the first!). The marriage was strategic, as his new wife, Bonadona 'sa Sala, came from a medical family; the archives document her two physician brothers practicing in Perpignan and Puigcerdá.[26] One of Abraham's marriages ended in divorce, but his career continued to thrive. He treated at least three of King Jaume II's children through the 1320s–1330s and was under contract as physician to the Infante Joan in 1339. He was also the physician for the count of Empúries, where he had a residence, and for the town of Castelló, the comital seat of Empúries, an independent territory adjacent to Besalú whose Jews were subject to the count, not the king.[27] In the early fourteenth century, an influx of moneyed Jewish immigrants to Empúries, some of them established lenders, created tensions with the longtime residents of the Jewish *aljama*. Whether Abraham's presence and residence in Castelló were part of this trend is unclear. Jewish physicians were highly over-represented in the bigger cities like Barcelona and Girona, and Empúries may have offered professional (and financial) opportunities scarcer in Catalonia.[28]

Even so, Abraham's ties with the royal court in Catalonia remained strong. In 1326, the same year that Abraham produced his study of simple humoral fevers called the *'Aleh Ra'anan* (*Fresh Leaf*), the king obligingly paid off some of the count of Empúries's debts to Abraham, granting the physician a thirty-year tax exemption inheritable by his daughter, Bonadona. Bonadona owed this tax break to the untimely death of Abraham's only son,

26 Michael McVaugh, *Medicine before the Plague: Practitioners and their Patients in the Crown of Aragon, 1285–1345* (Cambridge: Cambridge University Press, 2002), 59. Marie Kelleher, *The Hungry City: A Year in the Life of Medieval Barcelona* (Ithaca: Cornell University Press, 2025), 156, notes that infertility provided a legitimate reason for Jewish men to seek royal permission for a second wife; perhaps Abraham invoked this rationale.

27 "Ampuries" in the documents. See Stephen P. Bensch, "A Baronial *Aljama*: The Jews of Empúries in the Thirteenth Century," *Jewish History* 22, nos. 1–2 (2008): 19–51. Bensch describes the early fourteenth-century relocation to Empúries of wealthier Jews from Barcelona, Girona, and other Aragonese cities, in part to escape the crushing tax burdens on royal Jews.

28 Bensch, "A Baronial *Aljama*"; Elka Klein, *Jews, Christian Society and Royal Power in Medieval Barcelona* (Ann Arbor: University of Michigan Press, 2006). Kelleher, *The Hungry City*, 95 and n39, notes, "the reputation of Empúries as a notorious sponsor of pirates," particularly in the seizure of grain shipments during the famine years of 1333–1334.

Yahacel, who had died within the past year.[29] Other documents record payments from a widow in Empúries whose son Abraham had treated in 1325 but who also died. Interestingly, the king's gratitude specifies Abraham's service to the sick that year, hinting that a widespread disease event may have prompted Abraham's interest in humoral fevers.

Abraham's written legacy consists of three extant works. The *Tractate on the Spirit in Life*, the least known, survives in a single, late fourteenth-century copy; my sense is that this was an early composition, perhaps predating the other two.[30] Significantly, the role of the vital or animating spirit and the importance of individual humoral complexions and susceptibility to disease are topics that resurface in the later plague tractate. In addition to this work and the *Fresh Leaf*, we also have the treatise on pestilential and non-pestilential fevers presented here, and Abraham or his disciples assembled several practical compendia and recipe collections (one of the latter organized by disease for easy reference). The *Fresh Leaf* was his most popular work, and is extant in ten known copies, one under the anomalous title "A short treatise on all the putrid fevers";[31] the copies range from one fourteenth-century exemplar through the fifteenth century, in Sephardic, Sephardic-Provençal, Italian, and Byzantine hands. Citations of Abraham's therapeutic recipes appear in a physician's handbook along with Hebrew excerpts of plague tractates by Jean de Tournamire and Guillaume de Siliceto, and Estori haParhi's translation of the *Antidotarium Nicolai*.[32] Judah b. Solomon Nathan, a later fourteenth-century Jewish physician, cited the *Fresh Leaf* and incorporated some of Abraham's recipes into his own fever

29 In several manuscripts, Abraham is identified as the son of David and father of "the sage" Yahacel—a generic honorific that may or may not imply medical training. Evidence that descendants of this family were still in the area and practicing medicine survives in a brief reference to Jewish representatives from Girona who attended the Disputation of Tortosa in 1414; the source is cited by Yitzhak Baer and Ben Zion Dinur in their edition of the *Shevet Yehudah* (Jerusalem, 1947/48), 197, see the note to line 16: "From Girona came physicians from the Caslari family, Yahacel Bonjudah and Aa'[ron?] Bonj' the sage." I am grateful to Michael McVaugh for sharing archival attestations to Abraham's activities.

30 For the מאמר על הרוח הנמצא בחי (*Treatise on the Spirit in Life*), see Udine, Biblioteca Arcivescovile di Udine, MS ebr. 242, fols. 185b–204a. The work is miscatalogued in the National Library of Israel's KTIV database under "medical miscellany" (קובץ ברפואה).

31 The title is descriptive, as putrid fevers arise in the humours, but it is the only copy with this title.

32 St. Petersburg, National Library of Russia, MS EVR IV 109. The dated colophon attributes the copy (or the copy from which this copy was made) to Abraham Avigdor in 1424.

tractate.[33] Judah was a prolific medical translator and author working in the Montpellier orbit.[34] His own treatise on fevers is dated 1362, during the first major plague outbreak to follow the Black Death. There was good reason to be interested in pestilential fevers that year, and how recent authorities had understood and treated them. Judah b. Nathan's tractate thus also documents an active network of Jewish physicians across the Iberian-Occitan border who shared texts and ideas circulating among each other and among their Christian colleagues in Montpellier.[35]

Curiously, Judah does not cite Abraham's *Tractate on Pestilential Fevers and Fever Types*, but the earlier *Fresh Leaf* (which Judah calls the *'Aleh haRefu'ah*, the *Healing Leaf*), which never mentions pestilential fevers at all. Was Judah unaware of the later work, or did Abraham's insistence that the Black Death fevers were not pestilential sound embarrassingly mistaken by that second wave? The two extant versions of Abraham's plague tractate also raise this question, as we shall see.

Plague reached Catalonia in the spring of 1348 and was in Barcelona by the beginning of May.[36] By that year, Abraham was an established physician with a prestigious career in Besalú and neighbouring Empúries. His adamant insistence that the fevers he treated were not pestilential but humoral is defiantly presented as a minority view, although in fact several of his contemporaries shared his reservations about a pestilential diagnosis.[37] He further claims in his introduction that he felt it necessary to write

---

33 Most of the recipes are cited in the body of Judah's text; some were added as marginal notations by an unknown reader.

34 The family was rooted in Avignon. According to Renan, Judah's exact dates and residence are unknown, but Zunz thought he lived either in Avignon, Montpellier or Arles. Ernst Renan, *Écrivains juifs français du XIVe s.* (Paris: Imprimerie nationale, 1893), 228.

35 Luis García Ballester et al., "Jewish Appreciation of Fourteenth-Century Scholastic Medicine," *Renaissance Medical Learning: Evolution of a Tradition*, *Osiris* 2nd ser., 6 (1990): 85–117. Judah also cites Avicenna, Isaac Isra'ili, Bernard de Gordon, and Gilbert l'Anglais, the first two canonic to the Montpellier curriculum and the second two contemporary faculty and authors. On the "common medical culture of Languedoc and Catalonia," see McVaugh, *Medicine before the Plague*, 58.

36 Tzafrir Barzilay, *Poisoned Wells: Accusations, Persecution and Minorities in Medieval Europe, 1321–1422* (Philadelphia: University of Pennsylvania Press, 2022), 112. As noted above, plague seems to have entered the Iberian peninsula by at least two routes, not just the one Barzilay recycles from Benedictow; see Ole Benedictow, *The Black Death 1346–1353: The Complete History* (Woodridge: Boydell and Brewer, 2004); and for the two routes, see Oliveira da Silva, "Chronologies, Routes and Conditions."

37 Arrizabalaga, "Facing the Black Death," 237–88; see his comments on the treatises

to make his views known, as otherwise they would be forgotten. His belief that he stood alone in his assessment may express frustration at being ignored or testify to shattered networks of communication in a fraught time: pandemic disruptions affected the circulation of books and knowledge as much as they did people and other kinds of goods, and the exchange of ideas between Christians and Jews faced additional challenges. On the other hand, Abraham's fear that his opinions would be consigned to oblivion is a curious worry for a physician of his stature; nothing in Abraham's life or writings suggests timidity or self-doubt. But the debate among physicians was underway, and though his views had not swayed his opponents, he wrote to be on the record when time would prove him right.

Abraham disappears from the documentary records in 1349, perhaps a victim of the fevers he thought he could cure. There is no evidence that he had changed his mind about his Tractate's conclusions before he died, which makes the startling divergence in the two extant copies of the text more riddling. That is because one of those copies does revise Abraham's argument, reversing his diagnosis to endorse a pestilential diagnosis for the plague.[38] Beginning with a brief overview of the history of the plague tractate, let me then turn to *The Tractate on Pestilential Fevers and Fever Types*, how it has come down to us, and what other puzzles it contains.

The Plague Tractate

When Abraham Caslari decided to write his tractate on pestilential and other fevers, the genre was hardly fixed; it was born with the Black Death and solidified as a literary genre in the wake of that pandemic onslaught. Nonetheless, as historians of medicine have long recognized, the plague tractate was not invented *de novo* but owed its form and conventions to the popular health regimens, or *regimina sanitatis*, in circulation among medical professionals and their high-end clients—originally kings, popes, and high-ranking secular and ecclesiastical figures but increasingly members of an extended urban bourgeoisie.[39]

---

by Alphonse de Cordoba and the Montpellier Anonymous.

38 Reworking one's own compositions was common but unlikely in this case. See Diana Di Segni, "Gentile da Foligno's *Consilium contra Pestilentium* and Its Hebrew Translation," *Quaderni di Noctua* 7 (2024): 220, where she notes that "the rewriting and adaptation of contents is a typical feature of the literary genre of the Consilia." I see no reason not to extend the observation to the plague tractate, too.

39 Arrizabalaga, "Facing the Black Death"; Luis García Ballester, "Changes in the *Regimina sanitatis*: The Role of Jewish Physicians," in *Health, Disease, and Healing in*

Western and southern Europe of the late thirteenth into the fourteenth centuries were graced with the finest medical schools, faculties, and physicians anywhere on the continent, rivaled only by Italy's. Commissioned by anxious kings and municipal officials, their leading authorities began to produce writing about the fevers of 1348. Some of their responses targeted an audience of medically trained peers. Some were more practical, aimed at governments and bureaucrats. So, too, their languages varied. Arabic tracts were composed in Granada, the Maghreb, and the Middle East. In Christian territories, they tended to be in Latin, with rarer vernacular examples like Jacme d'Agramont's tractate for the municipal government in Lleida or the recently edited *aljamiado* tract published by Pilar Romeu Ferré.[40] Several early examples were written in the orbit of Montpellier or in Italy, and one was commissioned by the king of France from the medical faculty in Paris.[41]

For learned men of medicine, fever was not a symptom but a disease, defined as an alien or excess heat that threatened the heart. Categorizing different kinds of fevers was a major preoccupation of contemporary medical theory. Most fevers fell into one of three general categories: ephemeral or continuous fevers that arose in the pneuma (spirits), lasting only a day; putrid fevers that arose in the humours and might be intermittent (like malaria) or continuous; and hectic fevers, which began in a "member" (major organ).[42] Epidemic and pestilential fevers constituted their own category,

Medieval Culture, eds. Sheila Campbell et al. (New York: Palgrave-MacMillan, 1992), 119–31; Melissa Chase, "Fevers, Poisons and Apostemes: Authority and Experience in Montpellier Plague Treatises," *Annals of the New York Academy of Sciences* 441 (1985): 153–69; Lori Jones, *Patterns of Plague: Changing Ideas about Plague in England and France* (Montreal: McGill/Queen's University Press, 2022).

40 The term "aljamiado" refers to Romance vernaculars in Hebrew transliteration, often with elements of a uniquely Jewish dialect of that vernacular. See Pilar Romeu Ferré, *Tratado sobre la peste: Edición critica del manuscrito 2726 del Jewish Theological Seminary of America (siglo XV)* (Barcelona: Romanyà Valls, 2024). My deep thanks to Professor Romeu Ferré for sending me a copy of this work.

41 See Arrizabalaga, "Facing the Black Death," for a survey of the early exemplars.

42 Intermittent fevers included the quotidian, tertian, quartan; continuous fevers were either synochous, causon, or hectic. Lola Ferre, "Isaac Israeli's 'The Definition of Fever and its Essence' in its Hebrew Translations (The First Treatise of 'The Book on Fevers')," *Transactions of the American Philosophical Society*, n.s., vol. 111, no. 5 (2023): 1–256, at 91; Luis García-Ballester, "La recepción del Colliget de Averroes en Montpellier (c. 1285) y su inflencia en las polémicas sobre la naturaleza de la fiebre," in *Homenaje al Profesor Dario Cabanelas Rodriguez*, ed. García Ballester, vol. 2 (Granada: Universidad de Granada, 1987), 317–32; Demaitre, *Medieval Medicine: The Art of Healing, from Head to Toe* (Santa Barbara: Praeger/ABC-CLIO, 2013);

uniquely generated by putrefaction or corruption of the air that entered the body through respiration or even through the pores. Combinations of these "simple" (i.e., irreducible) categories were also possible, reflecting the real-world problem that what a physician was seeing did not always match what was in his books.

Like the popular health regimen, the plague tractate was organized into clearly defined sections, beginning with definitions, followed by causes, signs, symptoms, and treatment. Exposition unfolded within the framework of the Galenic six non-naturals to explain the humoral dyscrasia that could enhance or constrain a toxic putrefaction.[43] The non-naturals also determined the categories of recommended treatment (or prophylaxis). The **causes** of pestilential fevers might be celestial, such as eclipses or planetary conjunctions, or terrestrial, like earthquakes, floods, fetid water, rotting trees or crops, or wars that ravaged landscapes and left behind decomposing corpses.[44] Any of these things might corrupt the air, one of the four primary elements. The corrupted air then travelled to the heart, inflaming it with poisonous heat that was sent throughout the body. **Signs** included changes in the skies or climate, altered diet or behaviour that preceded the arrival of pestilence and were essential for recognizing it. **Symptoms** manifested the nature of the disease as it unfolded; and **treatments** were of two sorts, those that addressed the sick and those that addressed the healthy who wished to remain so. Depending on their target audience, a plague tractate might or might not conclude with recipes for various ointments, compresses, drugs, purges, and fumigations.

Chase, "Fevers, Poisons, and Apostemes"; Nahyan Fancy, "Medical Commentaries: A Preliminary Examination," *Oriens* 41 (2013): 525–45; Y. Tzvi Langermann, "Maimonides on Synochous Fever," *Israel Oriental Studies* 13 (1993): 175–98; Michael McVaugh and Linda Voigt, "A Latin Technical Phlebotomy Text and its Middle English Translation," *Transactions of the American Philosophical Society* 74, no. 2 (1984): 1–69; Carmen Peña Muñoz and Fernando Girón Irueste, "The Identification of Fevers according to al-Isra'īli, Avenzoar, and Bernard Gordon," *Cronos* 8 (2005): 95–120; Peter Pormann and Emilie Savage-Smith, *Medieval Islamic Medicine* (Edinburgh: Edinburgh University Press, 2007), 57–58.

43 The six non-naturals were defined as those factors that responded to conscious or inadvertent manipulation: climate or air; sleep and waking; food and drink; exercise; evacuation and retention; and mood. Demaitre, *Medieval Medicine*, 13; McVaugh, *Medicine before the Plague*.

44 Judah b. Nathan's fever tractate specifically indicates unburied corpses during wartime as a potential source of pestilence. New York, Jewish Theological Seminary Library, MS 2760.

Over the next few centuries, as plague outbreaks recurred, the plague tractate flourished. Historians of medicine have paid increasing attention to how they changed over time and in different settings. For a long time, modern discussions primarily focused on whether or when early physicians recognized contagion as a factor in the spread of plague. This focus was a distraction, not least because plague is not contagious, except in its pneumonic form.[45] Bubonic plague is a multispecies disease that relies on a cycle of transmission: bacillus to flea/arthropod to mammal. Most of the time, plague is not even a human disease: a spillover from a rodent colony moves it from wild to domestic mammals and then to humans. The modern obsession with contagion overlooked these facts, while implying that a precocious recognition of Black Death "contagion" was a rare insight of medieval physicians who braved the sclerotic ignorance of religious dogma.[46]

Early quarantine policies acknowledged that plague spread without understanding how. But in general, the modern fixation with contagion has blinded us to what mattered to medieval physicians and what *they* were seeing.[47] Abraham certainly saw a transmissible disease but that did not inter-

45 Ann Carmichael, "Universal and Particular: The Language of Plague 1348–1500," *Medical History Supplement* 27 (2008):17–52; Chase, "Fevers, Poisons, and Apostemes"; Lori Jones, "Bubo Men? Repurposing Medieval Anatomic Illustrations for Plague Therapy in the Fifteenth and Sixteenth Centuries," in *Death and Disease in the Medieval and Early Modern World: Perspectives from Across the Mediterranean and Beyond*, eds. Lori Jones and Nükhet Varlik (Woodbridge: York Medieval Press/ Boydell, 2022), 221–46; Jones, *Patterns of Plague: Changing Ideas about Plague in England and France 1348–1750* (Montreal: McGill-Queens University Press, 2022); Nükhet Varlik, *Plague and Empire in the Early Modern Mediterranean World: The Ottoman Experience 1347–1600* (Cambridge: Cambridge University Press, 2015); Varlik, "Four Colours of Disease and Death in the Early Modern Ottoman Cultural Imagination," in *Death and Disease in the Medieval and Early Modern World*, eds. Jones and Varlik (York: University of York Press, 2022), 123–48; Justin Stearns, *Infectious Ideas: Contagion in Premodern Islamic and Christian Thought in the Western Mediterranean* (Baltimore: Johns Hopkins University Press, 2011).

46 The famous example is Ibn al-Khaṭīb, the physician from Granada whose exasperated dismissal of religious *fatwas* prohibiting belief in contagion purportedly led to his assassination. As Justin Stearns, Mohamad Ballan, and others have shown, the courtier-physician-poet, for all his brilliance, was assassinated in 1374, years after the Black Death, in the wake of a failed diplomatic mission in the Maghreb. Mohamad Ballan, "Borderland Anxieties: Lisān al-Dīn ibn al-Khaṭīb and the Politics of Genealogy in Late Medieval Granada," *Speculum* 98, no. 2 (2023): 447–95; Stearns, *Infectious Ideas*.

47 Marilyn Nicoud, "À l'épreuve de la peste: Médecins et savoirs médicaux face à la pandémie (XIVe–XVe s.)," *Annales HSS* 78, no. 3 (2023), 508, also makes this point.

est him; he was focused on other things.[48] He also faced the challenge of writing in a language—Hebrew—that was poorly equipped to maneuver the concepts he needed to convey. The novelty of his formal approach, in which each section sequentially treats its subject matter (causes, signs, etc.) as it applies to pestilential, humoral-pestilential, and the recent fevers, captures the plague tractate at a moment when its conventions had not yet solidified. One of the two copies of the text, in turn, preserves an attempt to shift its argument by redirecting the tiered exposition to conform to a later consensus on the nature of the plague. To understand how that may have happened, we must look at the two versions carefully.

The *Tractate on Pestilential Fevers and Fever Types*

Abraham's opinion on the devastating fevers "of the past year" was, while not exceptional, unusual: he did not believe that the deadly fevers of 1348 were true pestilential fevers, but a different kind of fever triggered by environmental stress and famine.[49] He categorized these fevers as humoral with pestilential qualities. Because this view ran counter to the dominant view coalescing among his peers, his treatise took an unusual form intended to clarify his differences with his colleagues and underscore his own diagnosis. To this end, as noted above, the *Tractate on Pestilential Fevers and Fever Types* is uniquely constructed in parallel tracks that treat the definition, causes, signs, symptoms, and treatments in methodically alternating sections for true pestilential fevers, then humoral-pestilential fevers, and finally "the fevers of the past year."

This anomalous compositional structure, which has not been noted before, merits attention as a literary novelty, too. As an early illustration of a new genre, Abraham's tractate documents a moment before its conventions were fixed, and we can see him pushing boundaries that later would harden and close.[50] Like later exemplars, however, his treatise embeds state-

48 Like most of his contemporaries, he also shows no interest in the appearance of buboes as a plague symptom. The veins he recommends for bloodletting point to alleviation of swelling or abscess in the neck or groin regions, but he does not make this explicit. It may be that his focus on accumulated humoral putrefaction implied lymphatic swellings. Once again, his interest lay elsewhere.

49 Abraham will follow the conventional definition of a "true pestilential fever" as one caused by an alien (unnatural) heat due to a qualitative and poisonous change in the air; through respiration or via the pores, the heat enters the blood where it is carried to the heart and from the heart throughout the body.

50 Lola Ferre, "La terminología médica en las versiones hebreas de textos latinos,"

ments and interjections that alert us to the author's presence and illustrate the uses of authorial voice in medieval medical writings.[51] According to Marilyn Nicoud, the plague tractate allowed its author to assert expertise and authority, reinforcing physicians' status vis à vis "colleagues, patients and authorities."[52] I would put it more strongly and say that the plague tractate offered the physician-writer a literary means of self-fashioning that concentrated in the person of the physician an embodied performance of expertise, authority, and social concern. The tractates also testify to thriving networks of intellectual, professional, and social exchange that embraced a variety of healthcare workers from family members to barbers, surgeons, pharmacists, physicians, and even the later copyists who transmitted Abraham's work.[53]

In Abraham's case, we must also ask why and for whom he wrote in Hebrew, what kind of Hebrew he wrote, and what human and textual communities shaped his views. His combative assertions that unnamed colleagues had misdiagnosed plague patients, accordingly mistreating—and killing!—them, demonstrates a willingness to challenge a class of learned physicians who were products of the scholastic medicine taught in the universities, most notably and nearest in Montpellier. At least some of his unnamed rivals were Christians and university men; empirics would not have been invested in the texts or taxonomical distinctions he stresses. But Christian university physicians read Latin, not Hebrew: how would they encounter his critique? Learned Jewish physicians and students surely represented his immediate audience. From his other extant writings, we know Abraham maintained a robust presence among Jewish disciples and peers, and his wife was from a physicians' family with two brothers working in nearby towns. The wife of the contemporary satirist Maimon Galipapa in Lleida (presumably related to the chronicler) was licensed to practice medicine, but we have no idea if she or other women practitioners could read

---

MEAH, Heb. section, 40, no. 2 (1991): 87–107. Ferre's early article remains the only serious consideration of the tractate as a literary genre with distinctive conventions and stylistic features. See also James A. Secord, "Knowledge in Transit," *Isis* 95, no. 4 (2004): 654–72.

51 See Susan L. Einbinder, *Writing Plague: Jewish Responses to the Great Italian Plague (1631)* (Philadelphia: University of Pennsylvania Press, 2022) for treatment of this theme in early modern Hebrew plague writings.

52 Marilyn Nicoud, "À l'épreuve de la peste: Médecins et savoirs médicaux face à la pandémie (XIV–XVe s.)." *Annales HSS* 78, no. 3 (2023): 541.

53 Nicoud, "À l'épreuve de la peste," 511; Anna Collar, ed., *Networks and the Spread of Ideas in the Past: Strong Ties, Innovation, and Knowledge Exchange* (New York: Routledge, 2022).

Hebrew. Abraham had ample opportunity to interact with Jewish male and literate colleagues in Besalú, Empúries, and in service to the king and infante.[54] But was a disagreement with fellow Jewish practitioners, whose views leave no trace in larger debates, sufficient motivation for his tractate? Or was he working out an argument that he intended to reach farther?

Complicating these questions are the two extant copies of Abraham's treatise. Pinkhof based his 1891 edition on the copy in Leiden, Leiden University Library, MS or. 4778.[55] He was aware of the existence of a second copy in Paris, Bibliothèque nationale de France (BnF), MS héb. 1191, but felt that the Leiden text was more authoritative.[56] The following edition includes transcriptions of both sources with translations. Both copies were made in the fifteenth century and survive in large miscellanies of medical and philosophical texts, many of them medical works associated with the authors and curriculum of Montpellier's famous medical school. The Paris text is considerably shorter and often clearer, rephrasing Leiden's convoluted Hebrew as coherent, at times even elegant prose.

The peregrinations of Abraham's tractate over the century between its composition and these copies remain an unsolved mystery. The two copies clearly drew on different source texts. In some places, the difference shows up as stylistic or lexical; in others, the Paris manuscript has strikingly eliminated key passages in the Leiden copy, noticeably tamping down polemical passages in which Abraham expressed his disagreement with the unidentified colleagues who misdiagnosed as pestilence the fevers of the previous year. The biggest elision comes at the end of the treatise, where the Leiden text concludes with a chapter on "the fevers of the past year" followed by recipes for treating pestilential and humoral-pestilential fevers. The Paris copy has dropped the entire chapter on the last year's fevers, as well as the recipes for humoral-pestilential fevers, either in an attempt to refocus Abraham's diagnosis of the recent fevers on pestilence or because the categorization and treatment of a fever that had occurred a century earlier did not

54 For Abraham's wife, from the 'sa Sala family, see above. Jordi Font Estrela, "Las Sátiras misóginas de Maimón Gallipapa: 'El Voto de la viuda' y 'Querellas de una mujer,'" *MEAH*, Hebrew section, 44 (1995): 149–70; Eleazar Gutwirth, "En Maymon Galipapa: Texto y contexto de un intelectual ilerdense (s. XIV)," *Actes Ir. Colloqui d'Història dels Jueus a la Corona d'Aragó* (Lleida: Institut d'Estudis Ilerdencs, 1991): 339–48. For an old survey, see Joaquín Miret y Sans, "Les Médecins juifs de Pierre, roi d'Aragon," *Revue des études juives* 57, no. 114 (1909): 268–78.

55 Henceforth abbreviated "Leiden, MS or. 4778" or "Leiden."

56 Henceforth abbreviated "Paris, MS héb. 1191" or "Paris."

interest him. Certainly, by the time this copyist or his predecessor revised Abraham's text, he had seen plague return, perhaps more than once; physicians generally agreed that they were treating pestilence but also understood that not every epidemic had the same cause. Whatever his motives, the copyist's aggressive manipulation of the text reminds us that copyists played an active role in how texts "moved" over space and time, and in the debates they transmitted or altered.[57]

Abraham's 1326 treatise on humoral fevers, the *Fresh Leaf*, had launched the author's career as a learned physician, demonstrating his mastery of the Galenic categories and methods of university learning. The *Fresh Leaf* also documents Abraham's early interest in humoral fevers. Notably, it is a straightforward work that treats categories and treatments for simple humoral fevers and never mentions epidemic or pestilential fevers at all. What served as the catalyst for this early work Abraham does not say, but there are hints that he may have been motivated by an earlier disease event, perhaps even a precocious outbreak of plague. That episode could have been related (I speculate) to an attested disease outbreak in Pisa in 1324, while Aragonese forces battled their Pisan rivals for control of Sardinia.[58] The Black Death tractate occasionally echoes the *Fresh Leaf*, further implying that Abraham had noted similarities between the fevers of 1348 and an earlier event; those similarities would have fuelled his conviction that what he was seeing in 1348 he had already seen before.

Abraham follows the classical texts he had studied, from Galen to al-Isra'ili to Ibn Sina, defining a humoral fever as an excess of humoral matter, generating heat, in the organ that houses that humour or its nearby emunctories. That excess can have multiple causes, ranging from over-exertion to emotional turbulence to malnutrition. None of these factors, however, caused a *pestilential* fever, which depended upon a qualitative and poisonous corruption of the air that bypassed the humours to target the vital spirit in the heart before spreading throughout the body. Abraham insists that the

57 Secord, "Knowledge in Transit," 660–61.

58 Monica H. Green, "A New Definition of the Black Death: Genetic Findings and Historical Interpretations," *Medio Aevo* 11, no. 2 (2022): 139–55; Green, "Out of the East (or North or South)," 283–323; Philip Slavin, "Out of the West: Formation of a Permanent Plague Reservoir in South-Central Germany (1349–1356) and Its Implications," *Past & Present* 252, no. 1 (2021): 3–51. The Sardinian connection remains my speculation. For some background, see Mario Lafuente Gómez, "La conquista y colonización de Cerdeña por la Corona de Aragón: Historiografías nacionales, investigaciones recientes y renovación interpretativa," *Rivista dell' Istituto di storia dell' Europa mediterranea* n.s., 6 (June 2020): 105–45.

cause of the fevers that swept the peninsula in 1348 lay in the poor harvests and subsequent grain shortages that preceded them, forcing people to eat bread of pips and acorns. This combination of environmental and dietary stress was the catalyst for humoral dyscrasia that presented as a deadly fever; the extra toxicity of the fever gave it pestilential qualities. Enlisting the learning and experience of a long career, Abraham was sure that he was right. Scholars today who are interested in the confluence of famine and disease events may agree with him.[59]

The Manuscripts

The *Tractate on Pestilential Fevers and Fever Types* does not come down to us as a single document. While both copies clearly refer to the same source, their copyists must have had different versions of it. Leiden, MS or. 4778, the copy that formed the basis of Abraham Pinkhof's 1891 edition, is actually the later copy. The National Library of Israel's KTIV catalog dates the miscellany that contains the Leiden copy to the fifteenth–sixteenth centuries; the various texts that compose the miscellany are chiefly medical and in a variety of hands (Byzantine, Sephardic, and Oriental). The original catalogue entry in KTIV also indicated that there were two colophons, dated respectively to the Hebrew months of Nisan and Tevet 5244, corresponding to April 1484 and December 1483 of the Gregorian calendar. However, these colophons belong to the first section of the miscellany, which is unrelated to Caslari's treatise and is written in a different hand and Oriental script; the corrected entry now removes both colophons from the description of Caslari's text.[60] The Leiden miscellany runs over two hundred and fifty folios and has been haphazardly combined so that the component texts are sometimes missing heads or tails and shuffled randomly into place. Abraham's tractate is immediately followed by another, incomplete plague tractate by his near-contemporary, Abraham b. Solomon Hen.[61]

59 See below, 000 [for pagination at typeset proof stage].

60 The correction was made by Yael Okun at the Institute for Microfilmed Hebrew Manuscripts (IMHM) in the NLI following my inquiry, in May 2025.

61 Interestingly, the first colophon indicates that it was translated in the year of ה"ר'מ'ד', which seems to refer to one of the disease categories mentioned by Abraham that I could not identify. See Leiden, MS or. 4778, fol. 118b and Paris, MS héb 1191, fol. 118b. For the Hen text, see Bos and Mensching, "The Black Death in Hebrew Literature." Hen's tractate does not survive in entirety but discusses causes (celestial and terrestrial) then treatment or preventive measures organized with respect to the six non-naturals.

The second copy of Abraham's plague tractate, in Paris, MS héb. 1191, occupies fourteen folios in a huge miscellany of close to one thousand folios. This miscellany, much of it in Italian script, is dated to the fifteenth century. The binding is dated to the sixteenth century and bears the coat of arms of Henri II (r. 1547–1559), suggesting that the turbulence and local expulsions that characterized Jewish life in the south of France over this period may have parted an earlier Jewish owner from some or all of his library.[62] The compendium is an eclectic mix of philosophical, medical, astronomical, and religious texts, some of them translations (Aristotle, Hippocrates, Johannes de Leonardo), some classical Andalusian-Provençal texts (Ibn Gabirol, HaLevi, Ezobi) but also Jacob of Coucy's halakhic compendium, the *Sefer haMitzvot haGadol*, Maimonides' *Eight Chapters* and his commentary to the Mishnah. The medical selections are mostly practical and include both Abraham's *Fresh Leaf* and his *Tractate on Pestilential Fevers and Fever Types.*

The medical topics attested by both miscellanies emphasize fevers and pestilence, reflecting the deep interest of physicians in a disease phenomenon that had become a recurring feature of late medieval life. The non-medical hodgepodge of the Paris miscellany is a consequence of random binding, but it also reminds us of the durable mix of philosophical and metaphysical interests that shared intellectual space with scientific and, especially, medical knowledge.

The Leiden copy was destined for personal use: the hand is a hasty Sephardic semi-cursive, and the copyist made no attempt to produce a visually attractive work. The text is subdivided by headings written in larger "font" size, often embedded mid-paragraph. (I have indicated these with larger-font print in the transliteration and translation). In contrast, the Paris copyist cared more about an aesthetically pleasing result, his semi-cursive Sephardic script is neater and more regular, and his headings herald a new thematic section; they are written sometimes in larger semi-cursive script, sometimes in smaller, Rashi-style script. Perhaps this copy was commissioned for a personal library or by a fussier (or better-paid) copyist. Minimally, two types of reader are thus represented by the texts. Together, they tell us that among consumers of medical and philosophical learning, some but not all physicians, Abraham Caslari's tractate continued to circulate for over a century after his death.

---

62 See the BnF online catalog description at http://archivesetmanuscrits.bnf.fr/ark:/12148/cc8073s. My thanks also to Don Skemer, who confirmed the identification of the royal coat of arms in Marie-Pierre Lafitte, *Reliures royales du Department des manuscrits* (1515–1559) (Paris: BnF, 2001) 60n26.

Curiously, although the versions in the Leiden and Paris copies are often close, they can differ significantly. The divergences range from stylistic to strategic, the latter particularly evident in the Paris copy's deletions. The two extant versions retain the format of alternating sections on true pestilential fevers and humoral-pestilential fevers, but the Paris copy has vigorously suppressed much of the polemic that motivated the doubled exposition and with it the author's detailed treatment of the recent fevers. Both texts begin with the author's prologue, where Abraham explains why he has decided to write his tractate and for whom, and then they proceed in sequential "chapters" or sections. The skeletal outline of chapters follows:

Leiden	**Paris**
Introduction Definitions True Pestilential Fevers: – Causes: general; terrestrial; celestial – Signs – Prognosticating signs	Introduction Definitions Pestilential Fevers: – Causes: celestial; terrestrial – Signs – Prognosticating signs
Humoral-pestilential fevers – Signs & prognostication – Symptoms	Humoral-pestilential fevers – Signs and prognostication – Symptoms
Regimen for pestilence and true pestilential fever – Recipes	Regimen for pestilence and true pestilential fever – Recipes
For "unadulterated" pestilential fever – Recipes	Regimen for "unadulterated" pestilential fever – Recipes
Regimen for humoral-pestilential fevers – Recipes	Regimen for humoral-pestilential fevers END.
The fevers that occurred this year – Signs – Symptoms – Possible cause	
Regimen for the fevers of the past year – Recipes for purgatives – Recipes for ointments/plasters END.	

Even where its subject matter parallels Leiden's, the Paris copy downplays Caslari's preferred diagnosis of humoral-pestilential fevers, nonetheless preserving their regimen while eliminating treatment recommendations for pestilence. Both copies open with Abraham's description of the strange fevers that swept the region, baffling physicians and leading them to misdiagnose them as pestilential. In these excerpts, the texts are very close:

Leiden, MS or. 4778, fol. 115a–b

וכמעט שנעלמו מן הרופאים מיני הקדחות האלה ולגדריהם אותותיהם רבים ישפטום דבריים והנהיגום בהנהגת קדחות דבריות והיו משלחים להאכילם הבשרים כתרנגולים ויין לשתות בהתחלה והעלייה ולא יריקום והיו אומרים כי זה ראוי לדבריות. וראיתי שנהג זאת ההנהגה ומת. ויש שהיו מקיזים ומריקי' ומקיאים רב אלו היו נצולים וקצתם היו מתים לנפילת הכח.

> The types of these fevers nearly eluded the physicians, and their mixed signs led many to judge them pestilential, so that they treated them for pestilential fevers and would feed them meat like poultry and wine at the onset and during the increase, and not bleed them, as they said this was how to treat pestilential fevers. But I saw that he who followed this regimen died. Still, there were those who were bled and evacuated and purged greatly, and these were saved, [although] some died from loss of strength.

Paris, MS héb. 1191, fol. 135a

וכמעט שנעלמו מן הרופאים מיני הקדחות. רבים ישפטום דבריות וינהיגום בהנהגת קדחות דבריות עד שרבים מן הרופאים יאכילום הבשרים הדקים ובפרט בשר התרנגולים ויתירו להם היין בהתחלה והעלייה והתכלית ולא יריקום ויאמרו כי זה ראוי לדבריות. וראיתי כי רוב מי שנהג זאת ההנהגה מת. ויש שהיו מקיזי' ומקיאים ורובם היו נצולים וקצת היו מתים לנפילת הכח.

> The types of these fevers nearly eluded the physicians. Many judged them pestilential and treated them according to the regimen for pestilential fevers, so that many of the physicians fed them light meat, especially poultry, and they permitted them wine at the onset, increase, and duration and would not evacuate them, as they would say this was appropriate for pestilential fevers. But I saw that most of those who followed this regimen died. Yet there were those whom they would bleed and purge and most of them were saved, although a few died from loss of strength.

The Leiden copy retains Abraham's lengthy description of his goals in writing, a passage considerably truncated in the Paris copy:

Leiden, MS or. 4778, fol. 115b

ושאלו ממנו אנשים חכמים ונבונים שאודיעם סברתי בהנהגות הקד[ח]ות האלה ואכתוב בזה מאמר והשלמתי רצונם ויקובל תועלת כל חכם לכיוצא בחלאים האלה אם יקרו ויהיה התועלת להווים ויהיה המשל ודוגמא לבאים כמו שהם כל הספרים שחוברו בזאת המלאכה שהיא לפרטים שאין אחד וחליו שוה לאחד וחליו. ולכן אי אפשר שיהיו הנסחאות הפרטיות כתובות בספרים מאוזנות לפרטים הבאים אך יהיו כמדה ושקל ופלס לחכם יוסיף ויגרע לפי טוב שכלו וראיתי כי [אם] לא אודיע בברור הקדחות האלה מאי זה מין הם לא יפרסם אמתת סברתי בדרכי הנהגתם. ולכן כתבתי בקצרה מה ירצה באמרי דבר ודבר[י] בגדרים ואבאר סבותיהם ואותותיהם והנהגתם ואחר אודיע סברתי בקדחות האלה והנהגותיהם.

פרק הפלגתי לחשב בקדחות האלה ואותותיהם ואחשוב שאחזתי ענינים ולתועלת כללי כתבתי סברתי מאיזה מין הם ואיך תונהגנה. יעיין במאמר הזה מי שירצה יטה דעתו לדעתי או יטה ממנו או י[[ו]]סכם עם דברי או יחלוק עליהם האותות דרך ישרה לאמת.

Then wise and learned men requested I tell them my opinion for treating these fevers, and that I write this tractate. I fulfilled their wish and may any sage or such find it beneficial for these sicknesses if they occur. And may the benefit be for the present time and an example and model for those to come, as is the case for all the books that have been composed about this art, because it is concerned with individuals, for no man and his sickness is like another and therefore it is impossible that the individualized formulations written in books will be well tempered for future individuals. Let them be a measure and scale for the sage to add and detract according to his knowledge. I saw that if I did not clarify these fevers—what type they are—the truth of my opinion for treating them would not be disseminated. Therefore, I have written briefly what is meant when we say pestilence and pestilential, and their causes, signs, and treatment, after which I will make known my opinion about these fevers and their treatment.

CHAPTER: I thought intensely about these fevers and their signs, and I think that I have grasped matters that will serve the common good. I have written my opinion about what type they are and how they should be treated. Let the one who wishes study my tractate, whether he agrees or differs with my words or with respect to those signs, which lead directly to the truth.

Paris, MS héb. 1191, fol. 135a

ושאלו ממני אנשים חכמים ונבונים שאודיעם סברתי בקדחות האלה ודרך הנהגתם. וראיתי כי אם לא אודיע בבירור גדר הקדחות האלה ומאי זה מין הם לא יפורסם אמות סברתי בדרכי הנהגתם. לכן כתבתי בקצרה מה ירצה באמרנו דבר ודברי ואבאר סבותיהם ואותותם והנהגתם. ואחר כך אודיע סברתי בקדחו' האלה שקרו והנהגותיהם בע"ה.

פרק

אמר אברהם הפלגתי בקדחות האלה ואותותיהם עד שאחשוב שאחזתי עניינם ולתועלת כללי כתבי סברתי מאי זה מין הם ואיך תונהגנה. ומי שירצה לידע מה דעתי לפי סברתי ויסכים בזה או יחלוק עלי האותות יעשו דרך לאמת. ולהקדמה אבאר ואגדור שם הדבר.

> Then wise and learned men requested that I tell them my opinion of these fevers and how to treat them. I saw that if I did not make clearly known the definition of these fevers and what type they were, the truth of my opinion about their treatment would not be disseminated. Therefore, I have briefly written what is meant when we say pestilence or pestilential, and shall clarify their causes, signs, and treatment. Afterwards, I shall give my opinion about the fevers that occurred and their treatment, with the help of God.
>
> **CHAPTER**: Abraham said: I thought deeply about these fevers and their signs, until I think that I have grasped their matter, and for the common good, I write my reasoning about what type they are and how they should be treated. He who wishes to know my opinion, according to my reasoning, let him agree or disagree with me; the signs lead to the truth. For introduction, I will clarify and define the term pestilence…

In the Leiden copy, Caslari argues that the fevers of 1348 were *not* pestilential but a compound fever that occurs when "putrefaction in the spirit is taken up into the humours" (Leiden, MS or. 4778, fol. 116a). He calls this compound fever type humoral-pestilential and believes this is what he saw in 1348. His diagnosis is in part based on his observations but more importantly on what he understands to be the fever's cause.[63] The Paris text replaces the compound diagnosis with a discussion of simple humoral fevers, a fever category with no apparent relevance. But as we shall see, the distinction is critical, because a fever that is humoral in origin, with an

63 The proliferation of compound fever types, including humoral-pestilential, goes back to Avicenna, who describes a range of combinations in the *Canon*, Book IV fen 1.

added "poisonous" quality that gives it a pestilential aspect, demands a different treatment regimen from the treatment for pestilential fevers.

Indeed, Abraham has already expressed some frustration over the generic use of the term "pestilential" to include collective disease events precipitated by factors ranging from miasmic corruption to over-exertion or inadequate and irregular diets.[64] He will return to this last possibility towards the end of the Leiden copy when he asserts that malnutrition in the wake of crop failures may have been a "material cause" for the recent fevers:

Leiden, MS or. 4778, fol. 121a–b

ואפשר שהיתה סבת הקדחות האלה חמריות ר"ל מרוע הנהגת המזונות בכמותם ואיכותם כי היתה יוקר ומעט המצא מזונות הנאכלים הנהוגים בחמשת מיני התבואה ואכלו רוב העם לחם גרגרים וזרעים בלתי נהוגים חרצון וערמון ואלונים.

> The cause of these fevers may have been material, meaning bad dietary regimens, quantitative and qualitative. For there were high prices and shortages of the foods customarily eaten, the five species of grain, so that most people were eating bread [made from] kernels and seeds that they were not used to, fruit pips, chestnuts and acorns.

With this claim, Abraham emphasized a linkage that has kindled recent interest among historians of environment, climate, and disease. The connection between fourteenth-century climate change and its catastrophic impact on food production has been treated with growing sophistication in recent studies.[65] While the Great Famine years preceding the Black Death have been thought to have contributed to that pandemic's severity, the "bad years" did

---

64 Leiden, MS or. 4778, fol. 116a; Paris, MS héb. 1191, fol. 135b.

65 Interest has been catalyzed in part by our own climate crisis, but also by the unexpected resurgence of famines, predominantly in the Middle East and Africa. For the medieval period, bioarchaeologists Sharon DeWitte and colleagues have produced several studies examining the impact of famine and nutritional deprivation on susceptibility to disease and early mortality; see, for example., Sharon DeWitte et al., "Childhood Nutritional Stress and Later-Life Health Outcomes in Medieval England: Evidence from Incremental Dentine Analysis," *Science Advances* 11 (July 30, 2025), https://doi.10.1126/sciadv.adw7076. For more recent history, see the many studies of Alex de Waal: *Mass Starvation: The History and Future of Famine* (New York: Wiley, 2017); de Waal, "Memory and the Social Meanings of Famine," *Third World Quarterly* 45 no. 2 (2024): 439–43; de Waal, "Hunger in Global War Economies: Understanding the Decline and Return of Famines," *Disasters* 49 no. 1 (2024): https://doi.org/10.1111/disa.12661.

not disappear with the Great Famine's conclusion.[66] Catalonia was hard hit by famine in the mid-1330s and recurringly until the Black Death.[67]

Abraham describes the debilitating impact of malnutrition and predatory pricing on human immune systems.[68] His diagnosis—a humoral fever with pestilential qualities—reflects his focus on that causal chain. The distinction between his diagnosis and the pestilential diagnosis preferred by his unnamed colleagues carries through to their respective and antithetical treatments. For a true pestilential fever, where the humours are not involved, purging and bloodletting would be deleterious, evacuating good and necessary matter with the bad. In the case of humoral-pestilential fever, however, purging and bloodletting are essential, because the humoral excess must be removed. Abraham insists that he has vigorously purged and bled his patients, while his rivals have refused to do so and watched their patients die.

Abraham's methodical comparison of the two fever types in his treatise is thus polemical: having laid out his analysis of true pestilential versus humoral-pestilential fevers, he can turn to the recent fevers to show that they fit the latter category. That final step has been elided in the Paris copy. When the Leiden and Paris copies discuss the treatment regimen for unadulterated pestilential fevers, their language is fairly similar; in both texts, Abraham strongly warns against evacuative treatments of any sort

---

66 William C. Jordan, *The Great Famine: Northern Europe in the Early Fourteenth Century* (Princeton: Princeton University Press, 1996); the Great Famine was not as devastating in Catalonia as subsequent, recurring crises. For several recent studies focusing on this region, see Joan Maltas i Montoro, *Caresties, fams i epidemies a Catalunya: De la conquesta de Sicilia a la Pesta Negra* (Lleida: Pagès, 2022); Pere Benito i Monclus and Antoni Riera i Melis, eds., *Guerra y carestía en la Europa medieval* (Lleida: Editorial milenia, 2014); Adam Franklin-Lyons and Marie Kelleher, "Framing Mediterranean Famine: Food Crises in Fourteenth-Century Barcelona," *Speculum* 97 no. 1 (2022): 40–76; Susan L. Einbinder, "Drought and Plague in Fifteenth-Century Algiers: The Hymns of R. Simon ben Zemah Duran," *Medieval Encounters* (2026), forthcoming.

67 Kelleher, *The Hungry City*.

68 According to Michele Armstrong-Partida, powerful clerics were frequently implicated in price gouging for grain. Significantly, the longer-time resident Jews of Castelló d'Empúries, where Abraham provided medical care, were not highly urbanized; often holding small agricultural plots, they would have felt the impact of harvest failures and high prices quickly, all the more if they were involved in grain trade. Michele Armstrong-Partida, *Defiant Priests: Domestic Unions, Violence, and Clerical Masculinity in Fourteenth-Century Catalunya* (Ithaca: Cornell University Press, 2017), 94; Bensch, "A Baronial *Aljama*."

(purges, emetics, bloodletting), for fear that the evacuation will eliminate the pneuma, or spirit, along with the excess humour.[69] In no case should the patient be bled unless, in the physician's "balanced judgment," it is essential.

Both copies provide a regimen for treating humoral-pestilential fevers (although Paris eliminates the detailed drug recipes), and the Leiden copy concludes with recommendations for the fevers that recently occurred and that Abraham believes were likely humoral-pestilential. In the Paris copy, however, after the section on humoral-pestilential fevers, the tractate abruptly concludes. One possible explanation is that the copyist who made the original elisions wished to blur the argument that Abraham was making against a pestilential diagnosis; this would also explain why he stripped out or tamped down the polemical statements earlier in the text. Alternatively, the Paris text may have eliminated Abraham's concluding section on the "fevers that recently occurred" because by the copyist's time, they were neither recent nor relevant. In this reading, the Paris copyist was not interested in the historical question of what to call the fevers of 1348, but in the empirical question of what to do about subsequent fever outbreaks. He or his predecessor accordingly streamlined the tractate's contents to emphasize their continuing usefulness both for diagnostic and treatment options. Did this make Abraham's residual claims against a pestilential diagnosis less objectionable in hindsight? Where there was a consensus that the mid-fourteenth-century fevers had been pestilential, perhaps. Did the elisions reflect a later consensus that *subsequent* outbreaks were invariably pestilential? Not really. Rather, by retaining Abraham's discussion of humoral-pestilential fevers and their recommended treatment, the Paris text suggests that later physicians were aware that a new outbreak might be caused by different or compound diseases, not all of them bubonic plague.

For the historian, in contrast, it is precisely Abraham's discussion of the "recent fevers" that interests us. The text in Leiden gives explicit instructions for how to respond:

69 Leiden, MS or. 4778, fol. 120a; Paris, MS héb. 1191, fol. 140b.

Leiden, MS or. 4778, fols. 120b–121a

פרק בקדחות שקרו בזאת השנה. המאמ' הזה חברתיו ביחוד לבאר בהנהגת הקדחות שקרו בשנה הזאת ומקריהן ואותותיהן המשיגים והמפורסמים גם להמון וכ"ש לחכם רופא ולפי האותות לא יספק אחד מן החכמים כשאינן דבריות אמתיות שהוא תראינה באותות ומקרי הלחיית אלא אם יש ספק ישנו אם הם קדחות דבריות לחיות הנה לחות עלופיות לבד [[לבד]] להדמות אותותיהן המשיגים שהמצוקות והעלופים ירבו בליחות הדבריות ובליחות העלופיות בלתי דבריות. ומה שיבאר הספק הוא האותות המקדימות הלקוחות מתכונת האויר אם הוא דבריי אם לא ובסבות הדבריות אם קדמו. והנה לא נראו האותות באויר [[באויר]] באביב ולא בסתו ולא מערפליות ושאר ובריחת העופות מקניהן והרמשים מחוריהן. ולא נראה בפירות עפוש יותר מן העפוש הרגיל הטבעי להם. ואיך שיהיה הנה לחיים עלופיים שוה יהיה לחיים דבריים או לבד לחיים. וראוי שינהגו בהקזה או בהרקה אחרת לפי תגבורת הליחות המעופשות...

> I wrote this essay especially to clarify the regimen for the fevers that occurred this year, their symptoms and accompanying signs, which were evident even to ordinary people, let alone the sage physician. According to the signs, no sage would doubt that they were not true pestilential [fevers], because they appeared with the signs and symptoms of humoral [fevers]. If there was any doubt, it was whether they were humoral-pestilential fevers or merely fainting-humoral, whose accompanying signs look similar, for pain and fainting increase with humoral-pestilential [fevers] and with humoral-fainting [fever] that is not pestilential. What resolves the doubt are the prognosticating signs drawn from the form of the air and whether or not it is pestilential, and whether pestilential causes preceded [them]. Certainly, the signs in the air were not evident in the spring or fall, not in fogginess or the rest; the flight of the birds from their nests and the crawling things from their holes; the fruits did not show more rot than usual according to their nature. Howsoever it was, it's the same whether they were fainting-humoral or humoral-pestilential [fevers], or even just humoral: they should be treated with bleeding or some other evacuation according to the increase in the putrefied humours.

Abraham's insistence on bloodletting and other forms of purging for simple and compound humoral fevers remains intact in the Paris copy. In the Leiden copy, his insistence that the Black Death fevers were humoral-pestilential emphasizes his use of bloodletting and evacuations in his successful treatment of patients. Although Black Death physicians and their successors disagreed over the benefits of bloodletting for plague, Abraham was not alone in recommending this procedure, or even in rejecting a diagnosis of pestilential fever; rather, he participated in a larger debate over how to treat a seemingly novel and lethal disease. If we wait a short generation, his views would be echoed by several renowned physicians. Johannes Jacobi (d. 1384) also insisted that plague was a humoral fever of a more poisonous type. Guy de Chauliac (d. 1368) said it was not pestilential, and in Italy, so did Giovanni della Penna. Even Alphonse de Cordoba, who wrote during the Black Death, was not convinced that the Black Death was a true pestilential fever.[70] Abraham was not so much anomalous in his position as precocious. What effect phlebotomy had on Abraham's plague patients we cannot retrospectively know. What matters is that Abraham and a few of his colleagues discerned an effect that they attributed to this treatment, and that, locally at least, this assessment was rejected, much to Abraham's frustration.

The language of Abraham's *Tractate on Pestilential Fevers and Fever Types* also deserves comment. Abraham strove to demonstrate knowledge of the terminology and concepts that marked a learned physician. Like many efforts by contemporary Jewish physicians to convey in Hebrew the ideas they encountered in non-Hebrew texts and encounters, the results were uneven and their prose heavily dependent on loan words transcribed from Greek, Latin, Arabic, and Romance. Projecting knowledge and authority, moreover, does not improve Abraham's prose, testifying to the linguistic challenge of the Hebrew genre.[71] But here, too, we see differences in the two copies. The Hebrew of the Leiden copy can be especially challenging; by comparison, the Paris copy is almost elegant. The reader should keep in mind that my translations do not attempt to replicate contorted Hebrew but to make the Hebrew clear. I have tried to produce an English translation that

---

70 According to Chase, "Fevers, Poisons, and Apostemes," 157–59, the debate over definitions was intense between 1361–1381, when the plague returned twice.

71 The obscurantist style of the physicians was parodied in contemporary Hebrew belletristic works. For examples, see the excerpt from Qalonymos b. Qalonymos's *Even Bohan*, included as "The Physician," in Hayyim Schirmann, *HaShirah ha'Ivrit biSefarad uveProvanz*, 4 vols. (Jerusalem: Mossad Bialik and Dvir, 1956–1960) 2:510–14; and Maimon Galipapa's "Physicians' Aphorisms" in the same volume, 548–50 and 550–55. Galipapa's parody was published separately in *Shalosh Halatzot*, ed. Israel Davidson (New York, 1904); for an English translation, see Harry Friedenwald, *The Physicians' Aphorisms: A Medieval Hebrew Satire* (Baltimore, 1918), repr. from *Johns Hopkins Hospital Bulletin* 29, no. 325 (March 1918). Guy de Chauliac, slightly later, also spoofs the physician's arcane language. See Michael McVaugh, "Bedside Manners in the Middle Ages," *Bulletin of the History of Medicine* 71, no. 2 (1997): 201–23; Shem Tov Ibn Falaquera (d. 1290)'s "Epistolary Regimen for the Body and Soul" (in Hebrew) laments the limitations of Hebrew for expressing medical concepts.

faithfully represents what each version says, which also means that I have tried to render coherently passages that are less so in the original Hebrew. Whether the Hebrew text was corrupted by generations of copyists or whether it reflects the limitations of Abraham's Hebrew prose, the problem remains the same: in a real sense, I have sometimes distorted the Hebrew text by clarifying its meaning. That decision seemed justifiable in the interest of letting Abraham's reasoning and argument shine through.

Consider the following three examples. In the first, the two passages clearly express the same idea, but the Leiden text is comparatively awkward, laboriously claiming that the fact that a fever spreads (is transmissible) is not proof that it is pestilential, because changes in diet also cause sicknesses that alter the basic qualities of the air for non-pestilential reasons and spread. The sentence structure in the Paris text is much smoother, saying that transmissibility is not necessarily a sign of pestilence because it can occur in any sickness due to a change of diet from qualitative, non-pestilential causes.

Leiden, MS or. 4778, fol. 118a–b

ולא מהתפשטות הקדחות הרעות במקומות רבים ילקח ראיה על היותם דבריות כי אין התפשטות לחליים למזונות שנוי אנשי המקום מנהגם מזונות שלא היו רגילים בהם או זולתם מן הסבות באיכות חמים או קרים לחים או יבשים נתחדשו באויר מאיכות בלתי מעופש.

> And not from the transmissibility of the bad fevers over a great area is there proof that they are pestilential, because transmission of diseases from a change in local diet to unaccustomed foods and the like is not among the causes for qualities of heat, cold, moisture or dryness [to be] generated in the air from non-putrefactive qualities.

Paris, MS héb. 1191, fol. 138b

כי אין התפשטו' בחליים סגולה בדבריות כי ההתפשטות יהיה בכל החליים למזונות שינוי המקום ומנהג אנשיה במזונות שלא היו רגילים בהם או זולתם מהסבות באיכיות בלתי מעופש.

> That the fevers spread over a great area is not proof that they are pestilential, for the transmissibility of diseases is not a property of pestilence but occurs for all sicknesses [caused by] diet, change of location, and people eating foods they are not accustomed to and the like, from reasons [to do with] qualities that are not pestilential.

Sometimes, one copy (usually Leiden) drops phrases or words that are retained in the other (usually Paris) and that clarify a murky passage.

Leiden, MS or. 4778, fol. 117b

ולכן יהיה דפקי אלה ושתניהם קרובים לטבעיים עם היותם קרובים למות הגיעם ללב וקרבתם מהמות עד שלא יוכ הרופא להקדים הידיעה במותם מצד אותות השתן והדפק

> Thus, their pulse and urine will be close to natural even as they are close to death, as they reach the heart and they draw near to death, so that the physician cannot predict their death from the signs in the urine and pulse.

Paris, MS héb. 1191, fol. 137b

ולכן יהיו דפקי אלה ושתנים קרובי' אל הטבעיים עם היותם קרובים למות כאלו הם נשוכי או עקוצי הארסים שלא יראה ושלא יפרוסם שינוי ליחותם ולא יוכרו אותותיהם לפתאומיות הגיעם ללב וקירבתם מהמות עד שלא יוכל הרופ' להקדים הידיעה במותם מצד אותות השתן והדפק

> Thus, the pulses and urines of these people will be close to normal even as they are close to death, as if they were bitten or stung by something poisonous, because the change in their humours will not be manifested and their signs will not be recognized because of the suddenness with which [the poison-like spirit] reaches the heart, nor their imminent death. Thus, the physician is unable to predict their death from the signs in the urine and pulse.

Finally, in this third excerpt, the stylistic ease that characterizes the Paris text is less evident in English, but clearly so in Hebrew. The descriptive details preserved in Paris also offer a vivid glimpse of a medieval interior and its furnishings, illustrating the prophylactic importance of sealing liminal spaces like windows, thresholds, and the seams of paving stones with a sprayed or sprinkled barrier that is also used on the inhabitants' clothing.

Leiden, MS or. 4778, fol. 119a

ויריחו האנשים מאלה טבולים בחומץ ומעלה האתרוג ועשני נמאס הנקרא שרפול ויזו המקומות במים וחומץ ששרה בהם צנדליש כתוש ורדים והדס מ"א עשר חלקים לבונה חלק עלי אתרוג ועלי נמאס עלי אזוב מ"א שני חלקים ויוזה מהם המקום באויר הדבריי ויבואו במקומות האבניים וברכיים ובבתים הרצופים באבנים תחתיים מוזים בזה שקדם זכרו, וכ"ש בעת השינה שהכחות נרדמים ולא יחלקו על האיכיות הרעות הנשאפות כמו שיחלקו בעת התעוררם והיותם זריזות ובפועל.

> People should smell pomegranate leaves and the leaves of wild thyme called *serpoll* dipped in vinegar. They should sprinkle places with crushed sandalwood, roses, and myrtle steeped in water and vinegar—10 parts each; frankincense—one part; citron leaves, wild thyme leaves, and hyssop leaves—2 parts each; sprinkle

> them where the air is pestilential so they land on the stony and soft areas in houses paved with stone floors—sprinkle them with what we have mentioned before, and especially during sleep time when the faculties are dormant and will not oppose the bad qualities that are inhaled as they would when they are wakened and quick to actualize.

Paris, MS héb. 1191, fol. 139b

ויריחו עלי האתרוג וצירפוייל. ויזלפו המקומות במים וחומץ ששרה בתוכם צנדלי כתושים ורדים והדס מכל אחד י' חלק' לבונה חלק. עלי אתרוג עלי שירפוייל אנ" שני חלקים ויוזה מזה המקום אשר יעמדו בו ויושטחו יריעות בחלונות טבולות במים האלה וינעלו השערים. ויסתר האדים ממקום גבוה באויר הדבריי ויבואו במקומות האבניים ובספים ובבתים הרצופים באבנים מזולפים בזה. וכ"ש בעת השינה שאז הכחות נרדמים ולא יחלקו אל האיכויות הרעות הנשאפות כמו שיחלקו בעת התעוררותם.

> People should scent their clothing [by] dipping it in vinegar, and smell citron leaves and *serpoll*. They should sprinkle the area with water and vinegar steeped with crushed sandalwood, roses, and myrtle, ten parts each with one part frankincense; citron leaves, *serpoll* leaves—an oz., two parts each; and it should be sprinkled where they are, and curtains soaked in these waters should be spread [across] the windows and the shutters locked. [This] will destroy the vapours from high in the pestilential air; then they will descend to the stony places, the thresholds and the stone-tiled houses [that have been] sprinkled with this—[do this] especially when it is time to sleep because the faculties are dormant and will not oppose the bad qualities that are inhaled as they would when they are wakened.

Surprisingly, the recipes in the two copies are often remarkably close in ingredients and quantities. In some cases, ingredients have been added or subtracted, perhaps reflecting local experience, availability, or cost.[72]

---

72 In some cases, different languages describe the same herb, even at times in the same copy. Thus, for example, we find the Arabic *babunāj* and the Greek/Latin *camomila* in the same text. Likewise, the fever that Abraham identifies as frenesie (phrenitis) early in his treatise is referred to by its colloquial Arabic name, *birsām*, towards the end of the Paris copy. As Lola Ferre has noted, this linguistic instability is characteristic of the Hebrew treatises. Ferre, "La terminología médica." On the (mis)identification of phrenitis and *birsām*, see Nicola Carpentieri, Alexander Fidora, and Isaac Lampurlanés, "Avicena y Gerardo de Cremona sobre la frenitis: Una comparación entre al-Qānūn fī ṭ-Ṭibb y su traducción latina," *Al-Qanṭara* 39,

The yield of the recipes often exceeds what would have served a single patient, suggesting some compounds were scaled for a pharmacist to produce in quantity. Both copies refer to *materia medica*: a storage jar for a potion or electuary; silver and other vessels; red and white silk cloths for compresses; and a rich assortment of spices and minerals that would not be ordinary household items.[73] Among the therapies for humoral-pestilential fevers, both drugs and non-drug therapies like bloodletting, baths, compresses, or massage are prescribed for use over a period of days, indicating that patients might be expected to receive treatment for a week or so (accurate for bubonic plague).

Intriguingly, Abraham largely elided the sixth non-natural—mood, or affect—in his therapeutic recommendations.[74] The *Fresh Leaf* faithfully included the sixth non-natural in its prescriptive recommendations, urging the physician or caretaker to insure that the sick person refrains from "matters that agitate or worry [his] thoughts," instead taking him on walks with "companions and pleasant talk."[75] In contrast, the *Tractate on Pestilential Fevers and Fever Types* makes no such recommendation, even though Abraham has noted the plague patient's agitation and fear of death. His only concession to a patient's feelings or whims is to urge flexibility with the patient's diet, as the sick man or woman may crave a food that is otherwise not recommended. Abraham does not indicate why he ignored this regimen category. As noted above, he may have felt that the typical recommendations were impractical: pandemic conditions did not lend themselves to serene promenades and pleasant conversations, particularly If the patients were

no. 2 (2018): 293–320; Carpentieri and Taro Mimura, "Arabic Commentaries on the Hippocratic Aphorisms, vi.11: A Medieval Medical Debate on Phrenitis," *Oriens* 45, nos. 1–2 (2017): 176–202; Danielle Jacquart, "Les avatars de la phrénitis chez Avicenne et Rhazès," in Danielle Jacquart, *La science médicale occidentale entre deux renaissances (XIIe s.—Xve s.)* (Aldershot: Variorum, 1997), essay IX, 181–92; Fancy, "Medical Commentaries."

73 For the storage jar, see Leiden, MS or. 4778, fol. 119b and the corresponding passage in Paris, MS héb. 1191, fol. 140a. Maimon Galipapa's satiric *Physicians' Aphorisms* describes the profit-motivated collusion of a physician and a pharmacist, the former sending his recipes to the latter to compound and deliver to the patient; the physician urges him to take payment before handing over the medicine (implying its dubious odds of success). See Davidson, *Shalosh halatzot*. McVaugh, "El món medic de Castelló d'Empúries," 12, describes some of the botanical ingredients bought, sold, and compounded by local pharmacists.

74 Einbinder, *After the Black Death*.

75 Parma, Palatina Library (PL), MS Cod. Parm. Heb. 1952, fol. 6a.

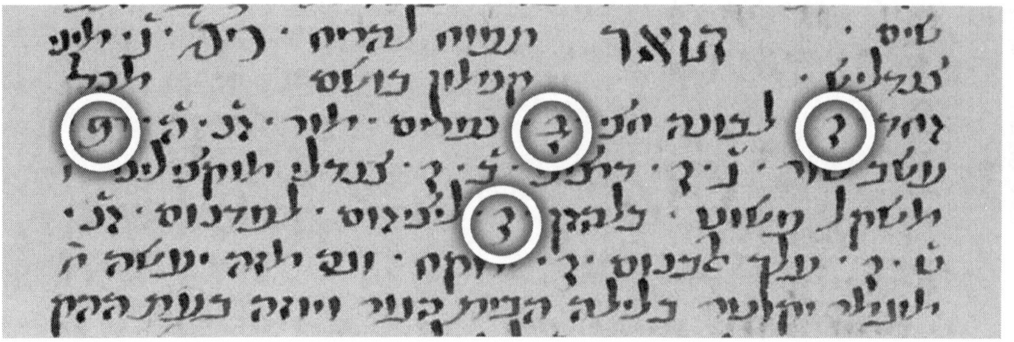

Figure 3. A close-up from the Paris copy of Abraham Caslari's plague tractate illustrating examples of the copyist's use of Latin or Greek pharmaceutical symbols to indicate weights and measures. Paris, Bibliothèque nationale de France (BnF), MS héb. 1191, fol. 140a. Reproduced courtesy of the BnF.

Jews fearing violence from their neighbours.[76] But why he would drop consideration of the patient's emotional state altogether is puzzling.

When recording recipes, the Paris copyist imported Latin pharmacological symbols for quantities and weights—drachma, scruple, ounce, and litra—directly into his text whereas they are transliterated into Hebrew in Leiden. Leiden also shows some preference for Romance quantitative measures—using the Hebrew אוק', for instance, for "ounce," as opposed to Paris's אונק', from the Latin "oncia."[77] In the Paris copy, drug (herb) names without Hebrew analogues are transliterated Latin, Greek, or Romance names, while

76 For a contemporary contrast, Abraham b. Solomon Hen's fragmentary tractate includes the sixth non-natural, urging that the patient's spirits be kept up. Bos and Mensching, "The Black Death in Hebrew Literature," 41. Einbinder, *After the Black Death*, wondered if Abraham's experience of dislocation, loss, and rebuilding encouraged suppression of past turmoil in his own life and less sensitivity to the suffering of others. I am unpersuaded by this argument now. Plague patients did not live long enough and were too sick for companionable strolls, while volunteers to accompany them were surely not abundant. Yet so many plague treatises refer to the dread and fear of death among the sick and their caregivers that Abraham's omission is curious. Whether the omission also implies an awareness that Jewish patients in settings that had experienced anti-Jewish violence were less likely to accrue any health benefits by hazarding a promenade is only my conjecture.

77 Di Segni, "Gentile da Foligno's *Consilium contra Pestilentium*," 235. Occasionally, Paris will also use אוק', so the copyist was not consistent. The same is true of the spellings for botanical ingredients, which can vary even in the same paragraph, a characteristic of the Hebrew treatises noted by Lola Ferre in an early study. See Ferre, "La terminología médica"; Di Segni, "Gentile da Foligno's *Consilium contra Pestilentium*," 237.

Leiden's drug names also assume familiarity with Arabic. For example, in a fumigant recipe:

Leiden, MS or. 4778, fol. 119a

ויריחו האנשים מאלה טבולים בחומץ ומעלה האתרוג ועשבי נמאס הנקרא שרפול

And people should smell from these dipped in vinegar and from citron leaves and the herb *nimās*, called *serpoll*.

Paris, MS héb. 1191, fol. 139b

שיריחו האנשים בגדים טבולים בחומץ ויריחו עלי האתרוג וצירפויי

That people should smell cloths dipped in vinegar, and they should smell citron leaves and *serpoll*.

Still, both versions use the Arabized כפור, כפר or כפיר for camphor, so this observation has exceptions. In other cases, differences in spellings suggest different languages or even dialects: Leiden's פירוניש for Paris's פרונש (plums), or Leiden's גראנט for Paris's גראנדש ([pome]granate), or Leiden's ארבאטור to Paris's עשב טור, perhaps again suggesting Leiden's (or Leiden's source's) familiarity with the Arabic *yarbaṭūra*, commonly called sulphurwort or sulphurweed in English. Scholars better equipped to identify these philological variants will find other examples as well. A handful of terms I am unable to identify.

Curiously, on the few occasions where the Leiden version embeds biblical phrases, which can bring with them rich associative connections that Abraham either consciously or unconsciously intended, the Paris copy sometimes dilutes or rewords them. The opening lines of both copies retain an allusion to Dt. 2:36, with its suppressed hints of anti-Jewish violence, but the Paris copy eliminates the allusion to Dt. 28:2's list of diseases that Abraham echoes to describe potential terrestrial causes of pestilence.[78] Abraham invokes Dt. 2:36, which describes the Israelite conquest of Canaan, but subtly inverts that verse's meaning to refer to the fever's ravaging "conquest" from Provence across Iberia. By linking the trajectory of the plague to a context of cascading violence, Abraham also ironically contrasts the biblical tale of Israelite triumph to their medieval helplessness.

Abraham's allusion to the diseases listed in Dt. 28:2 also adds leprosy to the biblical list. Not only does this tell us that contemporary Jewish

---

78 See Leiden, MS or. 4778, fol. 116b.

physicians accepted the prevalent association of leprosy with toxicity that could generate pestilential sickness. The inclusion of leprosy in Abraham's list also suggests the reverse: pestilential fevers could evoke leprosy and lepers, not only associated with disease but with the accusations and violence that had targeted them some twenty-five years earlier. In 1321, the so-called Lepers' Plot envisioned a conspiracy among lepers to poison Christian wells; according to the accusations, the lepers had been enlisted by the Jews, who were in turn acting on behalf of the Muslim "king" of Granada. Tzafrir Barzilay's recent study of well-poisoning libels assumed that the earlier episode had nothing to do with a disease outbreak, but if we are willing to push the appearance of plague in this region earlier, it certainly could have been a factor in earlier scapegoating of lepers and Jews, a memory echoing in Abraham's association of lepers and plague.[79]

In other examples, Paris eliminates the entire sentence where Abraham hopes that his tractate will be a "measure and scale" (Isa. 40:12) for future users.[80] And where in the Leiden copy, Abraham's treatment of the prognosticating signs for true pestilential fevers refers to the flight of "the dove, swift and crane" (Jer. 8:7), Paris has reworked the phrase to "types of crow, swift, and crane."[81] Lastly, although Paris has eliminated the entire chapter in which Abraham attributes the past year's fevers to harvest failures and irregular diet, the Leiden copy uses the rabbinic expression, "the five species," to refer to wheat, barley, spelt, rye, and oat; the faint link to the Deuteronomic curses that threaten failed harvests as punishment for Israelite disobedience has also been erased as well as any implication of environmental or political strains on health. Why the source text of the Paris copy swerved away from these intertexts is perplexing, but in so doing, it has also eliminated meaningful echoes in the biblical and rabbinic texts as well as the exegetical associations authors counted on their readers to know and enlisted as clues to local factors they preferred not to state explicitly.

Both copies avoid naming other authorities, living or dead. In general, medieval medical tractates loved to cite the authorities who bolstered their opinions or alternatively served as targets for refutation.[82] The *Tractate*

---

79 Barzilay, *Poisoned Wells*.

80 Leiden, MS or. 4778, fol. 115b; Paris, MS héb. 1191, fol. 135a.

81 Leiden, MS or. 4778, fol. 117b; Paris, MS héb. 1191, fol. 137a.

82 Again, Abraham b. Solomon Hen's contemporary tract does cite medical authorities, especially Hippocrates, al-Rāzī, Avicenna, and Galen's commentary on Hippocrates; see Bos and Mensching, "The Black Death in Hebrew Literature," 38.

on Pestilential Fevers and Fever Types refers pointedly to other physicians, invoking the "true physicians" or "true sages," the "wise physicians' books," or the "guild of physicians" whose judgments can be brought in support of Abraham's own opinions—but not a single one is named.[83] Proof that the choice was deliberate comes from Abraham's least-known and unexamined work, the *Treatise on the Spirit in Life*. Abraham concludes that work with his response to a student named Vidal, who has questioned Abraham's explanation of the relationship of spirit, humour, and member by citing the divergent explanation in Avicenna's *Canon*. Abraham's response opens with a preliminary discussion of why authors may choose not to cite the authorities they rely on or reject. One notable possibility is that the author may not wish to weaken his own argument by citing an authority who disagrees![84]

Nonetheless, we can see the traces of other authorities in the plague tractate. In the Leiden copy, Abraham concludes his chapter on the regimen for humoral-pestilential fevers by saying that he has abbreviated his coverage of this topic because it can be found in "the treatises and commentaries that all the great men of this art have written" (fol. 120b), which is a clever way of saying that those who are interested in this topic should read his own *Fresh Leaf*. His description of the prognosticating signs of pestilential fever is taken from Avicenna's *Canon*, which was circulating in Hebrew by the end of the thirteenth century.[85] So, too, his deference to the *Canon* is evident in his listing of fever types (fainting or phrenitis, for instance, but also the more familiar categories like hectic, causon, synochous, humoral, etc.). It seems highly likely that he is familiar with Bernard de Gordon's *Lilium*, which was

83 The same is true for the *Fresh Leaf*, which however Abraham indicates he wrote hastily over a three-day period. That cannot be his excuse with the later treatise.

84 See Udine, Biblioteca Arcivescovile di Udine, MS ebr. 242, מאמר על הרוח הנמצא בחי (*Treatise on the Spirit in Life*), fols. 202b–203a. Abraham breaks down his explanation into a set of categories including the deliberate suppression of cited authorities (what we would call plagiarism); original works whose author may or may not be aware of earlier works; and deliberate refusal to name an author whose arguments are being refuted.

85 Benjamin Richler, "Manuscripts of Avicenna's Kanon in Hebrew Translation: A Revised and Up-to-date List," *Korot* 8, nos. 3–4 (1982): 145*–68* (asterisks indicating the English section), 137–43 in Hebrew; Gad Freudenthal and Mauro Zonta, "Avicenna among Medieval Jews: The Reception of Avicenna's Philosophical, Scientific, and Medical Writings in Jewish Cultures East and West," *Arabic Sciences and Philosophy* 22 (2012): 217–87. Freudenthal and Zonta note that the *Canon* was one of a small handful of Avicenna's works enthusiastically endorsed by Jewish intellectuals in Iberia.

not yet translated into Hebrew but which Bernard had completed by 1304.[86] Certainly, the *Fresh Leaf*'s recommendation that a patient whose fever is accompanied by lethargy (or stupor) should be poked, pinched, have her hair pulled and be subjected to loud noises comes straight from Bernard.[87] Bernard also observed of pestilential fevers that a patient could exhibit no change in pulse or urine yet suddenly die, a formulation echoed in Caslari's plague tractate.[88] The recipe terminology suggests also that Abraham may have been familiar with the *Book of Simple Drugs* by Ibn Wāfid, translated into Hebrew by the thirteenth century.

Deliberateness may also lie behind Abraham's silence on the violence that assailed Jewish communities as near as Girona and Barcelona, rippling out across Aragon. On the one hand, a medical treatise is not the place to include social commentary. It is impossible that he was ignorant of the violence, whether he was treating victims who had fled the attacks, those who had attacked them (either of whom may also have been sick), or merely hearing second-hand reports. On the other hand, if I read his intended allusion correctly, his opening citation of Dt. 2:36 alludes to anti-Jewish violence.[89] Abraham's silence may be a strategic decision to avoid offending particular readers (although it is unlikely Christian physicians could have read a Hebrew work), or even a desire to block the memory of anti-Jewish violence. Alternatively, might the elision perform a wishful allegiance to a community of learned physicians—Christians and Jews—that he felt bestowed some immunity to the fate of his fellow Jews? This, too, is a mystery Abraham refuses to solve for us.

Medicinal plants posed another translation challenge, as there is no guarantee that the botanical names in the text truly correspond to the plants we know by those names. The violet offers an instructive example. Abraham

---

86 Na'ama Cohen Hanegbi, "Transmitting Medicine across Religions: Jean of Avignon's Hebrew Translation of the *Lilium Medicine*," in *Latin-into-Hebrew: Texts and Studies*, eds. Resianne Fontaine and Gad Freudenthal (Leiden: Brill, 2013), 1: 121–45. Jean's translation was completed in 1360, and a second Hebrew translation, by Yequtiel of Narbonne, in 1387. Cohen Hanegbi, "Transmitting Medicine across Religions," 126. Even in Besalú, Abraham could have had access to a Latin copy of this work. Michael McVaugh notes that a copy belonging to a Besalú apothecary was held in pledge by a Jewish lender in 1325: McVaugh, *Medicine before the Plague*, 90.

87 Demaitre, *Dr. Bernard de Gordon*, 154, and in the *Fresh Leaf* copy in Parma, PL, MS Cod. Parm. Heb. 1952, fol. 6b.

88 Demaitre, *Dr. Bernard de Gordon*, 64; also cited in Aberth, *Doctoring the Black Death*, 114.

89 Einbinder, *After the Black Death*, 79.

refers to this plant with the Romance term ויאולש ("*violes*") or ויאולט ("*violet*") in the plague tract and the *Fresh Leaf*, and indeed the violet is ubiquitous throughout Mediterranean medical writings, where it was enlisted for its purgative or astringent qualities.[90] Surprisingly, though, one of Abraham's recipes calls for stripping the violet of its "stems and thorns" (Leiden, MS or. 4778, fol. 120a, Paris, MS héb. 1191 fol. 141a). The plant we know as a violet has tender stems and no thorns. I first wondered if Abraham's "violet" must be a different plant from the one we call by that name, but concluded that he referred to garbling, the process of stripping the dried leaves or flowers from their stems or stalks. He simply had no Hebrew word for "garble."[91] In general, I have used familiar rather than scientific names for herbs and plants in the recipes; I know that this decision raises its own problems. Someone will surely find cause to emend some of the nomenclature.

Another intriguing botanical puzzle survives in one of Abraham's purgative recipes, which includes among its many ingredients the plant אשפרגס, like "violet" a transliterated name that clearly refers to "asparagus." The term appears in the Talmud, where it describes a strong botanical purgative, and it continues to find a place in post-rabbinic Hebrew medical recipes. It is not represented in Christian medical writings in Iberia, however, perhaps because the plant known as "asparagus" in Iberia is the vegetable we also call by that name, while the plant called "asparagus" in rabbinic sources refers to a plant in the same family but closer to what we call an asparagus fern.[92] Does the inclusion of "asparagus" in Abraham's recipe hint at familiarity with medical traditions beyond the Galenic medicine taught and produced in Montpellier? Were those traditions rabbinic? Salernitan? Empirical? This, too, remains an open but important question.

Where I have failed to identify the botanical or mineral substance to which Abraham refers, I have left a consonantal transliteration. Thus, for

---

90 See, for instance, the listing under ויאולש (violet) in a Hebrew pharmacological compendium from Portugal; the author or translator identifies himself or his father as originally from Leon and dates his copy to 1374. The manuscript is currently in St. Petersburg, Russian Academy of Sciences, Institute of Oriental Manuscripts, MS C 21; the digitized copy in the KTIV database is cross-listed by their microfilm number F 69263. Violets, listed on fol. 145b, are warm in the first degree and beneficial for a variety of digestive ailments, some fever-related.

91 I decided to volunteer with an herb farmer and did some garbling. The stems and parts of the dried flowers and herbs do become sharp and spiky, and I was advised to wear gardening gloves. My thanks to Christina Dedora, Cheryl Dedora-Pynn, and Kathy Taylor at Sanctuary Farm Herbs in Cranston, RI, for taking me in and teaching me.

92 Alan Cooper, email message to the author, July 2025.

example, מנא נאר is transcribed simply as MNA NAR (Leiden, MS or. 4778, fol. 122a). Hopefully, other readers will identify the missing terms in the future.

* * *

In sum, a comparison of the two copies of Abraham's *Tractate on Pestilential Fevers and Fever Types* sheds light on the life of this work after Abraham's life, and on the evolving debates over the nature of the fevers we call plague, as well as on the professional reputations that rose and fell with those debates. The two versions offer opportunities for comparison in addition to those I have included, some in the domain of philologists and scholars of medieval pharmaceuticals, some among historians of medicine interested in theory and therapeutics, and some among historians of the Black Death who may hopefully integrate Abraham's observations into the archival, historical, paleogenetic, and archaeological evidence of the Black Death's impact in the Besalú region. The way that the Paris copy routinely reformulates and improves the Hebrew of the Leiden copy also deserves greater attention. If, as it seems, different source texts were the models for the two versions, when did they diverge? Is it possible that Abraham originally composed a vernacular draft of the tractate that was subsequently rendered into Hebrew by two different translators? Alternatively, did the Paris copyist himself, or one of his predecessors, intervene stylistically to improve a Leiden-related version of the text, along the way aggressively editing and eliding to suppress what seemed in retrospect an erroneous diagnosis? Or does the editorial revision that survived in the Paris copy attest rather to the disinterest of later readers in the historical episode we call the Black Death and a shifting focus to the author's empirical recommendations as they might apply to current outbreaks?

Whatever we learn about these matters in the future, we can already see that the Paris copy of Abraham's plague tractate reveals a rapidly changing consensus on what the plague was and how to treat it. Abraham wrote his *Tractate on Pestilential Fevers and Fever Types* to prove to his colleagues that the Black Death fevers of 1348 were not pestilential fevers, but a compound type of humoral fever called humoral-pestilential. The latter emerged, not because of astronomical or terrestrial causes associated with pestilential alterations in the air, but as a consequence of poor harvests and high prices leading to scarcity and malnutrition. These crisis conditions had forced hungry people to consume unaccustomed foodstuffs, encouraging their susceptibility to humoral fevers that took on a poisonous or pestilential quality. The treatment for these fevers demanded relief of humoral excess by means of bloodletting or other types of evacuation. Significantly, even when the Paris version elides this discussion, it leaves his therapeutic recommendations intact, suggesting that fifteenth-century physicians saw multiple explanations for the epidemic fever outbreaks they witnessed and treated: some were pestilential and some not, some were compound and some simple, some unadulterated and some syndemic. They were sharp observers.

Over his lifetime, Abraham Caslari's prestige as a physician, like his personal wealth and status, left many archival traces, each of which offers a glimpse into the legal and financial dealings that accompanied the professional medical activity of a prominent physician. In all three of Abraham's surviving treatises, the *Fresh Leaf*, the *Tractate on the Spirit in Life*, and the *Tractate on Pestilential Fevers and Fever Types*, he states that he writes at the request of admirers or disciples. As a primer on humoral fevers, the *Fresh Leaf* is offered to readers who are eager to practice medicine but lack essential knowledge; the *Tractate on the Spirit in Life* is also addressed to students or disciples. Whether a literary topos or historical fact, these assertions place Abraham in a social, professional, textual, and teaching community that included a range of learned and less learned men who shared an interest in the medical debates, theories, and yes, crises, of their day.

Did Abraham succumb to the very fevers he claimed success in treating? The records of his activities go silent after 1349. He would not be the only learned physician who weighed in on the Black Death and did not live to reconsider his opinion; Jacme d'Agramont in nearby Lleida also died of plague after completing his treatise, as did Gentile da Foligno in Italy. As Guilleré showed years ago, physician mortality in the Girona region was relatively high compared to other professions; so was the mortality rate for notaries, textile merchants, barbers and surgeons.[93] Whatever the cause of Abraham's death, it makes it unlikely that reshaping his plague tractate was his own idea. Indeed, from what we can deduce of Abraham's character from the testimony of the archives and his own writings, he was not the kind of man to change his mind. When a later hand intervened, perhaps in the wake of the 1361–1362 recurrence, or following a subsequent outbreak, it was the hand of someone who knew and admired the author and wanted his work to last, perhaps not so much as a historical witness but a practical guide to pestilential recurrences. His intervention was characterized by editorial scrubbing that attests to the ongoing debate about the nature and treatment of plague.

93 Christian Guilleré, "La Peste noire à Girone," *Annals de l'Institut d'estudis gironins* 7 (1984): 87–161 at 121.

In Hebrew, Abraham's plague tractate also responded to non-Jewish texts and authorities who had something to say about the fevers of the Black Death. If a subsequent editor found it advisable to tone down his acerbity, he did not entirely erase the impatient self-assurance of a major Jewish physician disagreeing with his peers. In closing this introduction, and leaving the texts to speak for themselves, I want to underline how much this tractate projects an image of its author along with its medical argument. This ultimately literary act of self-fashioning presents the physician's voice as a verbal extension of his weight and meaning in a social world. For Abraham, authorial voice amplifies the place of personal rivalry and combative debate in the circle of medical authorities he knew and admired. By the same token, other voices—including that of the copyist who reframed his argument—also sound as we read the competing versions of this text.[94]

When the Paris version of Abraham's tractate was modified by a later editor, the debate was mostly over. In contrast, Abraham was writing a new kind of literature in the immediate aftermath of unprecedented crisis; the choices he made convey the urgency of the moment and the passion of the professional men who tried to stem the force of a pandemic. Subsequent generations of Jewish physicians sustained a dialogue with that passion and the texts that embodied it. Finally, if we take him at his word, most of Abraham's patients lived. His tractate still guards the mystery that might definitively tell us why, in our terms, that was so. But that is only one of the questions this work raises that still need answers. We still have much to learn from Abraham b. David Caslari and the physicians, surgeons, and healers with whom he agreed or disagreed. Collectively, these men and women did what they could in the worst pandemic of recorded history, they struggled to apply knowledge and skill to serve a common good, and sometimes, surely, they healed. Equally movingly, they also thought about what their experience might offer for future pandemic encounters. In other words, they wrote for us, too.

My transcription of the two Hebrew texts follows, in facing pages, and then my English translations followed by Hebrew-English and English-Hebrew glossaries. A brief description of method, format, and abbreviations precedes presentation of the texts.

---

94 Carpentieri and Mimura, "Arabic Commentaries on the Hippocratic Aphorisms," 176, note that the commentary genre has been undervalued as a means of self-expression and debate. I extend their observation to the work of the copyists, whose work also treads on exegetical and polemical ground.

Tractate on Pestilential Fevers and Fever Types

The Hebrew title מאמר בקדחות דבריות ומיני הקדחות appears only in the Paris copy of the text. The Leiden copy is untitled. I present the texts below in facing transcriptions to facilitate comparison; for discussion of the differences between the two versions, see the preceding introduction.

When the copyist has struck out a word or phrase either by crossing it out or inserting elision marks, I have transcribed the word or phrase then indicated its intended deletion with a line through it. Where I have added a word or phrase to clarify meaning I have enclosed it in single brackets. Dittographies are indicated with double brackets around one instance of the doubled word.

For the English translation of the Leiden copy, in addition to the manuscript folio, I have indicated the pagination for the 1891 Pinkhof edition, on the assumption that some readers will want to check it against my transcription. Please remember that Pinkhof only used the Leiden manuscript and that his transcription is occasionally inaccurate. Note also that because his transcription appeared in a Dutch publication, his pagination runs backwards, beginning with page 51 and concluding with page 39.

As noted in the introduction, plant names I was unable to identify are transcribed in the translations as consonantal transliterations in capital letters. Biblical citations are indicated with bold font, and so are chapter headings. For subsection headings, which both copyists signalled with larger script, I have used capitalized letters in larger font. Where the Paris copyist especially has also enlisted Rashi script for a subsection marker, I have used italics.

Abbreviations

Biblical and rabbinic citations use conventional abbreviations, e.g., Deuteronomy, chapter 2, verse 36, is abbreviated Dt. 2:36 in English, דב' כ:לו in Hebrew. B. Ketubot 79b refers to the Babylonian Talmud (versus a Y prefix for the Jerusalem Talmud), Tractate Ketubot, page 79b, and so on.

Weights and measures: The copyists do not employ consistent abbreviations for quantities or measures. As noted in the introduction, the Leiden text suggests a preference for Romance terminology, the Paris for Latin. For ounce, accordingly, we find the abbreviation אוק' in Leiden and אונק' in Paris; I have translated both as "oz." For dram, the Hebrew usually appears as the abbreviated דר'; I have used the full term or "dr." in the translations. For litra, both Leiden and Paris abbreviate with ל'; again, I have retained the full word.

The basic units of measure are the scruple, dram, ounce, and pound; Caslari uses litra frequently also. The value of these units varied a bit from country to country; Ronald Zupko's helpful article[95] lists the precise (or imprecise, as the case may be) apothecary values for England and France. Approximately, a scruple (from the Latin *scrupulus*) is about 1⁄24 ounce; a dram (from the Greek *drachmē*) is 3 scruples or 1/8 ounce; an ounce (Latin *uncia*, Romance *onca*) is 8 drams or 24 scruples; a pound (Latin *ponda*, but synonymous with *libra*, Romance *litra*, hence the abbreviation "lb.") is approximately 372 (English) or 367 (French) grams or twelve ounces. Paris, interestingly, sometimes (but not always) lists measures using pharmaceutical symbols. The following symbols will be used to denote key measurements: ℈ for scruple; ʒ for dram; and ℥ for ounce.

The Paris copy is held in the National Library of France, indicated as BnF (Bibliothèque nationale de France). The National Library of Israel is abbreviated NLI; within the NLI, the Institute for Microfilmed Hebrew Manuscripts, which manages the KTIV database of microfilmed and digitized manuscripts, is abbreviated IMHM.

Notes to the Hebrew transcriptions chiefly indicate my emendations, citations of biblical or rabbinic text, or other comments relating directly to the Hebrew. The fuller notes to the English translations include explanatory commentary or bibliographic sources as I thought helpful. Full citations for works cited in the English translations may be found in the bibliography.

---

95 Ronald Zupko, "Medieval Apothecary Weights and Measures: The Principal Units of England and France," *Pharmacy in History* 32 no. 2 (1990): 57–62.

The Texts

TRANSCRIPTIONS AND TRANSLATIONS

LEIDEN, LEIDEN UNIVERSITY LIBRARY
MS or. 4778, fols. 115a–123b

[115א]

אמר אברהם קשלרי הערני לחבור הזה מה שקרה בקיץ וסוף האביב כללו פרוונצה וקטלניאה ווילינצייה ומחוז אריגאון וקצת נאברי וקשטילה לא היתה קריה ועיר ששגבה מקדחות וכ"ש הדמיים טובי ה[נ]הגה.[1] והיו קדחות חדות המתים ממנה לא יעברו הי"א ורובם מתו בא'[2] ובז' והיו הקדחות תמידיות ובלתי פוסקות רבות העלוף והמצוקה ונפילת הכח. מהן שהתחילוה ברתת חזק וזיעו זיעה גדולה וחזקה ביום הראשון ואחרי הזיעה תתחזק הקדחת ותשאר מתמידה. ויזועו בשלישי ובחמישי והם מתמידות וגם בז' יזועו עם חוזק המצוקה רבים מתו במצוקה. ורבים עלו החמרים אל הראש עם פרנשין ובלבול השכל. ורבים מוצו או יקרם רפיון האיברים וימותו יקרם רעיפת הדם מנחיריהם רב מאד ובנשים דם הנדות ורבים יקרם קיא ושלשול חזקים או הקזה או הקיאו או שולשולו ברפואות ונצולו רבם ממי שקרה להם אחת מההרקות האלה או יותר אם ישמור כחם כראוי. וכ"ש שנצלו אם יהיה ההקזה או הקיא או השלשול בהתחלה. ורבים יצאו מהם תולעים אחר השלשול והקיא ונצלו או בשלשול ויציאת התולעים מן המצוקה והעלוף והיו אותות הקדחות מבולבלי' ברבים[3] מן המוקדחים. ולפעמים יתראו מקרי הדם באודם הפנים ולפעמים מקרי הלבנה בתרדמה ואסטוטות[4] ולפעמים מקרי האדומה בתעורה וצמא ונגוב הלשון. ושתני רבים מהמוקדחים ביום הא' זך ממי דק ואחר יתעבה ויתאדם ולהם כאב הראש חזק. ויש שיתלבן שתנ[[א]]ם פתאום אחר היותו ימים עכור ואדום ומפני שהיו פתאומים וחדים לא ייחלו לאיש ולמלאכת רופא מהמיתה וכמעט שנעלמו מן הרופאים מיני הקדחות האלה ולערבוב אותותיהם רבים ישפטום[5] דבריים והנהיגום בהנהגת קדחות דבריות והיו משתלחים להאכילם הבשרים כתרנגולים ויין לשתות

[115ב]

בהתחלה והעלייה ולא יריקום והיו אומרים כי זה ראוי לדבריות. וראיתי שנהג זאת ההנהגה ומת. ויש שהיו מקיזים[6] ומריקי' ומקיאים רב אלו היו נצולים וקצתם היו מתים לנפילת הכח.

ושאלו ממנו אנשים חכמים ונבונים שאודיעם סברתי בהנהגות הקד[ח]ות האלה ואכתוב בזה מאמר והשלמתי רצונם ויקובל תועלת כל חכם לכיוצא בחלאים האלה אם יקרו ויהיה התועלת להוים ויהיה המשל ודוגמא לבאים כמו שהם כל הספרים

---

1 בכת"י "הגהה."

2 השווה פאריס: עדיף לקרוא "בה' ובז'."

3 בכת"י "ברקים."

4 לתקן לקרוא "אסטניסות" כמו הנמצא בכ"י פאריס.

5 בכת"י "יפשטום."

6 בכת"י "מזיקים."

DOI: 10.17302/dohf20856 © Arc Humanities Press, 2026

PARIS, BIBLIOTHÈQUE NATIONALE DE FRANCE
MS héb. 1191, fols. 134b–141a

[134ב]

מאמר בקדחות דבריות ומיני הקדחות

אמר בן השלם דוד אברהם בנו אבי החכם יחצאל הקשלרי העירני לבבי לחבר המאמ' הזה במה שקרו בקיץ וסוף האביב קדחות כללו כל מחוז פרוינציאה וכל קטלונייאה וארגון לא היתה קריה ששגבה מהקדחות וכל שכן בבחורי הדמיים טובי ה[נ]הגה והיו הקדחות ההם ממיתות אותם לא יעברו אחד עשר יום ורבים ימותו בה' וז' והיו הקדחו' בלתי פוסקות רבות העילוף והמצוקה. מהן מי שיתחיל ברתת ובחום חזק ויזיע החולה זיעה חזקה ביום הראשון ואחר הזיעה תחזק הקדח' ותעשה מתמידה. ויזיעו בג' ובה' והנה מתמידות גם בשביעי יזיעו עם חוזק מצוקה ורבים מתו במצוקה. ורבים מהם עלו החמרים על הראש עם פרינישין ובלבול השכל. ורבים שימצו ואז יקרם רפיון האברים וימותו. ורבי' יקרם רעיפת דם הנחירים רב מאד ואל הנשים הגרת הנדות או קיא או שלשול חזק הוקזו והקיז ושולשלו בתרופו' ונצולו רבים ממי שקרה להם אחת מההרקו' האלה ויותר אם ישמר כחם כראוי. וכל שכן שנצולו אם היה בהם יציאת הדם או קיא בהתחלה או שלשול. ורבים יצאו מהם תולעים אחר השלשול ויציאת התולעים מן המצוקה והעילוף. והיו אותות הקדחו' מבולבלים ברבים מהמוקדחי'. ולפעמים יתראה מקרה הדם באודם הפנים. ולפעמי' מקרה הלבנה בתרדמה ואסטניסות. ולפעמים מקרה

[135א]

האדומה בתעורה וצמא ונגוב הלשון. **ושתני** רבים מהמוקדחים ביום ראשון ושני זך מימיי דק. ואחר יעבה ויתאדם ויעכר. ולהם כאב ראש חזק. ויש שיתלבן שתנם פתאום אחר היותו עכור ואדום. ומפני שיש מהם פתאומים וחדים לא ייחלו לאיש ממלאכת הרופא מהמית[ה] וכמעט שנעלמו מן הרופאים מיני הקדחות. רבים ישפטום דבריות וינהיגום בהנהגת קדחות דבריות עד שרבים מן הרופאים יאכילום הבשרים הדקים ובפרט בשר התרנגולים ויתירו להם היין בהתחלה והעלייה והתכלית ולא יריקום ואמרו ~~זה~~ כי ראוי לדבריות. וראיתי כי רוב מי שנהג זאת ההנהגה מת. ויש שהיו מקיזי' ומקיאים ורובם היו נצולים וקצת היו מתים לנפילת הכח.

ושאלו ממני אנשים חכמים ונבונים שאודיעם סברתי בקדחות האלה ודרך הנהגתם וראיתי כי אם לא אודיע בבירור גדר הקדחות האלה ומאי זה מין הם לא יפורסם אמות סברתי בדרכי הנהגתם. לכן כתבתי בקצרה מה ירצה באמרנו דבר ודברי.[1] ואבאר סבותיהם ואותותם והנהגתם. לאחר כך אודיע סברתי בקדחו' האלה שקרו והנהגותיהם בע"ה.

1 דבר ודברי – כתוב עם נקוד בכת"י

DOI: 10.17302/dohf20857 © Arc Humanities Press, 2026

שחוברו בזאת המלאכה שהיא לפרטים שאין אחד וחליו שוה לאחד וחליו. ולכן אי אפשר שיהיו הנסחאות הפרטיות כתובות בספרים מאוזנות לפרטים הבאים אך יהיו במדה ושקל ופלס לחכם יוסיף ויגרע לפי טוב שכלו וראיתי כי [אם] לא אודיע בברור הקדחות האלה מאי זה מין הם לא יפרסם אמתת סברתי בדרכי הנהגתם. ולכן כתבתי בקצרה מה ירצה באמרי דבר ודבר[י] בגדרים ואבאר סבותיהם ואותותיהם והנהגתם ואחר אודיע סברתי בקדחות האלה והנהגותיהם.

פרק הפלגתי לחשב בקדחות האלה ואותותיהם ואחשוב שאחזתי ענינים ולתועלת כללי כתבתי סברתי מאיזה מין הם ואיך תונהגנה. יעיין במאמר הזה מי שירצה יטה דעתו לדעתי או יטה ממנו או י[[ו]]סכם עם דברי או יחלוק עליהם האותות דרך ישרה לאמת.

יש שיקראו דבר או דבריי כל מין מחלה מתפשטת בעיר או מחוז או מחוזות והיא ממיתה מי שקרהו ולא יבדילו בין מי שיהיה ממנו בסבת אויר נשתנה איכותו לאחד מן האיכיות יחדש מחלה או מחלות מתפשטות[7] לסבות יגיעות ועמלות עשו אותם אנשי הבית או עיר או מחוז או לקיחת מזונות רעים או מרבים

[116א]

על בלתי מנהג לקחום אנשי העיר או מחוז או מחוזות יחדשו מחלה מתפשטת ביושביהם ובין מחלה מתפשטת להפסד אויר ועפושו כאלו הוא ארסיי ויקראו כל המינים האלה דבריות. **ואמנם** המיוחד בשם דבר או חולי דבריי שנאמ' עליו שם דבר ביחוד ובהסכמה הוא קדחות מתפשטות בסבת אויר מתאייך בעפוש והפסד לה כארסיי יעפש הרוח האנושי ויגיע העפוש פתאום אל הלב בשאיפת האויר התמידיית הבאה ומתערבת עם רוח הלב מהרה

ויתחמם ויוליד קדחות מתמידות להתמיד העפוש ברוח וזה העפוש וההפסד אפשר שיהיה בבית אחד או חלק ממנו ואפשר שיהיה העפוש וההפסד בחלק גדול מן הארץ עיר או עיירות או מחוזות ואקלימים ולא יתחדשו החליים האלו כי אם למוכנים השוכנים במקומות ההם ותהיינה רבות ההמתה מהרה תהיינה רבות המצוקה להיות הרוח אשר בלב מעופש אע"פ שלא יתפשט העפוש אלא ברוח וכשיהיה כן כמעט שלא ישתנה השתן מטבעו שנוי בליחה. ולא בדפק שנוי גדול ולא יהיה באחד מן האיברים כאב מצד הקדחת אלא יקרה להם שהשתן והדפק יהיו קרובים לטבעם והחולה כבר נטה למות בסבת הפסד רוח הלב שהיא קרוב לנפש שהיא סבת החיי ואם אולי התלקח העפוש מן הרוח לליחות או למקצתן בסבת שכנות הרוח וערובו בליחות ותתהוינה קדחות בסבות עפוש הליחות והרוח אז תהיינה הקדחות ליחיות דבריות לא דבריות ועם אותות קדחות ליחיות בדפקים והשתנים והכאבים. ושנוי פעולות הכחות המיוחדות באבר אשר הליחה בו ולפי הליחה שנתעפשה.

אם במוח והיתה דמיית יתאדמו הע[י]נים וירבה הכובד בראש ותעורה תרדמית עם בלבול בדמיון ומחזה תמונות אם היתה במוקדם המוח. או בלבול השכל והמחשבה אם בחדר האמצעית או היזכרות שכחיי אם היתה

[116ב]

7 בכת"י "מתפשטת."

פרק

אמר אברהם הפלגתי בקדחות האלה ואותותיהם עד שאחשוב שאחזתי עניינם ולתועלת כללי כתבי סברתי מאי זה מין הם ואיך תונהגנה. ומי שירצה לידע מה דעתי לפי סברתי ויסכים בזה או יחלוק עלי האותות יעשו דרך לאמת. ולהקדמה אבאר ואגדור שם הדבר.[2]

יש שקראו דבר לכל מחלה ממיתה פתאום

[135ב]

מתפשטת בעיר או מחוז או מחוזות. ויש הבדל בין ההתפשטות להפסד אויר לעפוש ובין מה שיהיה ממזונות רעים או בסבת יגיעות ועמלים היוצאים ממנהגם התמידיי בזמן הקודם וחודשו בהם בסבת זה הקדחת.

ואמנם המיוחדות בשם קדחת הדבר הם קדחו' היה סיבתם אויר נתאייך בעפוש ר"ל מצד קלות התפעלותו משכונת נבלות ופגרים גם משכונת עשבים ואילנות אשר בייחוד טבעם מעפשים האויר עפוש דבריי. כגון התאנה והאגוז והכרוב וכ"ש כשעליהן נופלין ונובלים. גם משכונת מימות נבאשות ומים מכונסים ומשרת פשתן אשר כל אלה רושמים באויר רושם מעופש יעפשו הגופות אשר יוכנו לקבל אותו ההפעלות וההפסד בחום ולחות ועפוש. והרוח האנושי מצד התערבו בשאיפת האויר התמידיי עם הרוח אשר בלב יתחמם אז ויוליד קדחת מתמדת להתמדת העפוש ברוח. וזה העפוש וההפסד אפשר שיהיה בבית אחת או בחלק אחד ממנו ולא יתחדשו חליים כי אם לשוכנים בבית ההוא. ואפשר שיהיה העפוש וההפסד בחלק גדול מן הארץ עיר אחת או עיירות ואז יהיה חלי הדבר בשוכני המקום ההוא המוכנים לזה. ותהיינה הקדחות ההם רבות המצוקה להיות הרוח אשר בלב מעופש אע"פי שלא נתפשט העפוש בליחות כי אם ברוחות וכשיהיה כן כמעט שלא ישתנה השתן מצבעו הטבעי לפי שאין שנוי בליחה. וגם הדפק לא ישונה שינוי גדול ולא יהיה שם כאב באחד מן האברים. ובאלה יקרה שהשתן והדפק יהיו קרובים לטבעם

[136א]

והחולה כבר נטה למות בסבת הפסד הרוח אשר בלב שהוא כלי קרוב לנפש שהוא סבת החום. ואם אולי התלקח העפוש מן הרוח אל הליחות או למקצתם בסבת שכונת וערבוב הרוח בליחות ותהיינה הקדחות בסבת עפושם והפסדם אז תהיינה הקדחו' ליחיות בשתנים ובדפקים והכאבים ושינוי פעולת הכחות המיוחדות באבר אשר שם הליחה שנתלקח בה העפוש ולפי האברים שיהיו בהם הליחה יהיו המקרים ולפי הליחה שנתעפשה. **דמיון** זה אם היתה במח והיתה דמיית יתאדמו העינים ויבלטו הפנים ויתאדמו וירבה הכאב בראש ותעורה תרדמיית עם בלבול בדמיון אם היתה במוקדם הראש ומחזה התנומות או בלבול בשכל ובמחשבה

---

2 דבר – כתוב עם נקוד בכת"י

בחדר המאוחר. ואם היתה דמית באצטומ' והכבד יקולקל הכח המאוה והמעכל ושאר הכחות העובדים לכח הזן. וכן יתקלקלו הכחות ~~העובדים~~ לפי עפוש לחה ולחה באבר ששם הליחה שנתעפשה וכבר כתבו זה חכמי הרפואה האמיתים בחבוריהם שם ימצאנו כל חכם לב ואין מכוון לזה המאמר כי לא כוונתי אלא לבאר איך יונהגו המוקדחים בעת המקרה שקרה בזאת ההנהגה וכל עת ומקום שיקרה כמוהו אלא שהביאנו זה הנה לבאר הקדחות שקרו.

הקדחות הדבריות האמתות אשר בעפוש אויר תמידי רב וכאלו הוא ארסיי באויר בשאיפתו יתעפש רוח הלב ויתחמם חום זה מעפוש רע ארסיי מבלתי שיתעבר לליחות שוה תהיה באיש אחד או שמתפשטת באישים.

סבות הקדחות האלה הסבה הכוללת היא עפוש האיור בחום ולחות נכרי המקיף במקום מה יהיה כולל וחלק כולל מאקלים או אקלימים או יהיה מקום פרטי עיר אחת או בית אחת או חלק מהם מאי זה סבה שיהיה העפוש. וסבות העפוש הם ארציות או שמימיות. והארציות יהיה משכונת העפושים מפסידים האויר בשכונת בעלי הגדמות והצרעת והנשדפים והחרחורים המתעבר הפסדם לאויר והפעולות. ויהיה לשכונת חליים רבים וגם מחלאים בלתי מתעברים. ויהיה לשכונת עשבים [[עשבים]] ואילנות אשר ביחוד טבעם מעפשים האויר עפוש דבריי לפי מה שהסכימו עליו המנסים והמקשים. וכן יראה בבחירה כתאנה ואגוז וכ"ש בעת נפילתו נבלת עליהם והפסדם. ויהיה לשכונת מימיות נבאשות ויאורים וחריצי מים ואגמים מקבצים נפסדים ומשרת פשתן וזולתו.[8] ויותר אם יהיו הדברים נבלות בעלי חיים ארסיים ועשבים בעלי איכות רע ארסיי

[117א]

ארסיי ויתפש ההפשט במרחק גדול או קטן מן העולם ויחזק או יחלש לפי רוב ומיעוט וחוזק וחולשה וארך וקצר והמשך ההפסד הוא המעפש האויר ולפי הכנת המקומות לקבול

~~והנהגה~~[9] [והסבה] השמימיית הוא שיתעפש האויר בזמנים מה הבלתי שכונת דברים ארסיים מעפשים בסבת שמימיית הרצון לחול כוכב מן הכוכבים המזיקים בערך אלינו במקומות מן הגלגל שגזר השם י"ת להשפיע שפעים מזיקים בערך

להויתנו ומזגנו ואם אמנה כי כל מעשה השם[10] טובים בעצמם ובערך לכלל המציאות. ובהיות הסבה עפוש האויר סבה שמימיית תהיינה הקדחות המתילדות בסבתו חזקות והמיתה פתאום מהתעלמות המקרים מסבות הקדמות ידיעת הרופאים מבלבלות שכלם באיכות הנהגתם לסובליהם לפי דעת הכוכבים ומקום מבטיהם וסבותיהם עד שלא יובן ענינם והנהגתם והקדמת ידיעת תכליתם כי אם לבעלי משפטי הכוכבים אותם שהתבודדו[11] באמות הסבות השמימיות ההם שהזדמנה.

---

8 השווה כ"י פאריס ע' 135ב.

9 לתקן לקרוא "הסבה."

10 ברור שכוונתו ל"מעשי השם טובים". הטעות מעלה את האפשרות שהמעתיק עבד עם מכתיב ולא ממדגם כתוב.

11 לתקן לקרוא "שהתבוננו" לפי כ"י פאריס.

ואם הליחה דמיית באצטומכה ובכבד יקולקל הכח המאוה והמעכל ויתר הכחות העוברים לכח הזן וכן יקולקלו הכחות לפי עפוש ליחה וליחה באבר ששם הליחה שנתעפשה. **וכבר** כתבו זה חכמי המחקר האמתיים בחבוריהם שם ימצאנו כל חכם ואין ביאורנו מכוון במאמר זה שלא כוונתי בו כי אם לבאר איך ינהגו המוקדחים בעת המקרה שקרה להם בשנה הזאת ויועיל ג"כ בכל עת ומקום שיקרה כמוהו לפי האותות הנזכרים למעלה

פרק

קדחת הדבריית האמיתית היא אשר בעפוש אויר תמידיי רע וכאלו הוא ארסיית באויר בשאפיתו יתעפש רוח הלב ויתחמם חום זר מעופש רע מבלתי שיתערב לליחות שוה תהיה באיש אחד או שתהיה מתפשטת באישים. ***סבות הקדחו' האלה***

[136ב]

הסבה הכוללת היא עפוש אויר בחום ולחות נכרי מקיף במקום מה שיהיה כולל חלק גדול מאקלים או אקלימים או יהיה מקום פרטי כמו עיר אחת או בית אחת או חלק מהם באיזו סבה שיהיה העפוש. ***וסבות העיפוש הם גם ארציות גם שמימיות.*** **הארציות** יהיה משכונת בעלי הגדמות והצרעת והנשדפים המתערב הפסדם באויר לקלות התפעלו ויהיה ג"כ לשכונת הנבלות והפגרים וגם לשכונת הרעבים שנשימתם מרוח נפסד. והיה ג"כ לשכונת עשבים ואילנות אשר בייחוד טבעם מעפשים האויר עפוש דבריי לפי מה שהסכימו עליו בעלי הנסיון והמקישים. וכן יראה בשכונת התאנה והאגוז והכרוב בעת נפילת עליהן והפסדם. ויהיה ג"כ לשכונת מימות נבאשות ויאורים וחריצי מים ואגמים מקובצים נפסדים ומשרת פשתן וזולתו. ויותר אם יהיה הדברים נבלות ובעלי חיים ארסיים ועשבים בעלי איכות רע ארסיי ויתפשטו ההפסד במרחק גדול או קטן מן העולם או יחלש לפי רוב ומיעוט וחוזק וחולשה ואורך וקוצר המשך ההפסד ההוא המעופש המעפש האויר וכפי הכנת המקומות לקבול

השמימיית היא שיתעפש האויר בזמנים מבלתי שכונת דברים ארציים מעפשים.

סבות שמימיות הרצון בזה לחול כוכב מן הכוכבים המזיקים בערך אלינו במקום ממקומות הגלגל שגזר השם י"ת בהם להשפיע שפעים מזיקים למזג האדם והרעיל אותו. או לחבור כוכבים מזיקים ישפיעו שפעים מרעילים

[137א]

האויר רעים בערך להוייתנו ומזגנו ואם אמנה כי כל מעשה השם טובים בעצמם ובערך בכלל המציאות ובהיות הסבה לעפוש האויר סבה שמימית תהיינה הקדחות המתילדות בסבתה חזקות והמיתה פתאומית נעלמות המקרים מכאיבות מכחישות הקדמת ידיעת הרופאים מבלבלות שכלם באיכות הנהגתם לסובליהם לפי דעת הכוכבי' ומקום מבטיהם וחבוריהם עד שלא יובן עניינם והנהגתם והקדמת ידיעת תכליתם כי אם לבעלי משפטי הכוכבים אותם שהתבוננו באמות הסבה השמימיית ההיא בהזדמנה.

פרק באותות הקדחות האלה אותותיה המשיגים מצוקת הלב החזקה לא בסבת כאב שאין תגבורת ליחה ה[ו]רגש וחום מתלהב עם עפריות מראה ונפילת הכח המנהיג פתאם כמי שילאה מתנועה ושירגיש בעצמו בחולשה עד שידמה הוא וכל המונו שהוא צריך למזון ודעיכת החום הטבעי לרוח מצד שהכחות כולם נשואים ברוח כשתדעכנה הרוחות יחלשו הכחות הנשואים בהם ובדחיות הכח החיוני המניע המיוחד בלתי תהיה יגיעה ולאות באברים. ורוב מה שיקרה להם נפילת התאוה למאכל ובלבול השכל לדעיכת הרוח אשר במוח המשתלח אליו מהלב גם את הרוח הוא במוח מעצמו מבלתי שיביאהו

[117ב]

מהלב כמו שיסברו כת מהרופאים ויקרם פחד ואימות מות. ולא יטה השתן מעצמו ומראהו הטבעי דבר רע שאין שם תגבורת ליחה ואיפשר שישתנה שנוי מה במקרה תעורה יקרהו או צער או עמידה מאכילה. ולא ישתנה

הדפק השנוי המתחייב לתגבורת ליחות יוצאות מן השווי באיך או בכמה אך אפשר שיתחלפו השתן והדפק התחלפות המתחיב להפעליות נפשיות מנטיית הרוח מהשווי. ולכן יהיה דפקי אלה ושתניהם קרובים לטבעיים עם היותם קרובים למות הגיעם ללב וקרבתם מהמות עד שלא יוכל הרופא להקדים הידיעה במותם מצד אותות השתן והדפק ~~התחייבות המתחלף להפעליות~~[12] וגם לא מקצת מקרים אחרים ממקרי הגוף הטבעיים.

פרק באותות המקדימות לחליים האלה אמנם מה שסבתם אויר נפסד בסבת דברים ארציים מפסידים הסבות ההנה הנה אותותיהם. ואמנם הקדחות הדבריות אשר בסבת שמימיות מאוירות בהפסד שיראה האויר קודם קרות החלאים מעורבב ערפליי בחום זר מצוק הלב כשישאף כאלו הוא חום עשן עצים לחום עב. ועלי הצמחים יותקו ויפלו קודם זמני נפילתם. והפירות יתעפשו מהרה והבעלי חיים יברחו מקנם שהבורא י"ת הטביע בבעלי חיים הרגשת האוירים הטובים וברח מהאוירים הרעים הנפסדים וביחוד קצת מיני העופות כעורב ומינו **ותור וסיס ועגור**. וכאשר יראה האותות האלה יוכל הרופא להקדים הידיעה שהקדחות תהיינה דבריות.

ואולם בעלי משפטי הכוכבים ידעו זה מצד משפטי הכוכבים בעת חבורי הכוכבים והלקיות ומשפטי העתים כמו שהוא מבואר בחכמה ההיא. וזה אין לרופא מצד שהוא בעל מלאכת הרפואה לדעת זה שחכמת הרפואה לא תעבור אלא הדברים המקובלים מבעלי חכמת הטבע והדברים הידועים

[118א]

[[הידועים]] בחכמת הרופאה. אותותיה הסגולים והמיוחדים התמדת השתן והדפק היות טבעיים או קרובים לטבעיים והמצוקות רבות מבלי הראות תגבורת ליחה באצטומ' או זולת מהאיברים אך שאר האותות הנזכרים באותות המשיגים בקדחות האלה הנה תמיד יקרו לקדחות הליחיות.

---

12 מסומן כטעות בכת"י.

פרק באותות הקדחות האלה

אותותיה המשיגים מצוקת לב חזקה לא בסבת כאב שאין שם תגבורת ליחה. וירגיש חום מתלהב עם עפריתיות המראה ונפילת הכח המנהיג פתאום שילאה מהתנועה ושירגיש בעצמו חולשה עד שידמה הוא וכל המזגי' שהו צריך למחזק ודעיכת החום הטבעי לרוח ומצד שהכחות כולם נשואים ברוחות כשתדעכנה הרוחות יחלשו הכחות הנשואיים בהם. ובייחוד הכח החיוני המניע המיוחד אשר בלב. ותהיה יגיע' וליאות באברים. ורוב מה שיקרה להם נפילת התאוה למאכל ובלבול השכל לדעיכת רוח אשר במוח המשולח אליו מהלב. או גם אם הרוח ההוא מעצמו מבלתי שיבואהו

מהלב כמו שיסברו כת מהרופאי' ויקרם הפסד ואימת מות. ולא יטה השתן מעצמו ומראהו הטבעי דבר רב לפי שאין שם תגבורת ליח' ואפשר שישתנה שינוי מה שבמקרה יקרהו תעורה

[137ב]

או צער או עמידה מאכילה, וגם לא ישתנה הדפק השינוי המתחייב לתגבורת ליחות יוצאות מן השווי באיך או בכמה. אז אפשר שיתחלפו השתן והדפק התחלפות המחייב להפעליות נפשיות ולנטיית הרוח מהשווי . ולכן יהיו דפקי אלה ושתניהם קרובי' אל הטבעיים עם היותם קרובים למות כאלו הם נשוכי או עקוצי הארסים שלא יראה ושלא יפורסם שינוי ליחותם ולא יוכרו אותותיהם לפתאומיות הגיעם ללב וקירבתם מהמות עד שלא יוכל הרופ' להקדים הידיעה במותם מצד אותות השתן והדפק ולא מקצת מקרים אחרים ממקרי הגוף הטבעיים.

פרק *באותות המקדימות לחליים האלה*

אמנם מה שסבתם אויר נפסד בסבת דברים ארציים מפסידים האויר הסבות ההם הנה אותותיהם. ואמנם הקדחו' הדבריו' אשר יתהוו מסבות שמימיות מאיכות האויר בהפסד הוא שיראה האויר קודם החליים מעורבב ערפלי וחום זר מציק כשישאף כאלו הוא עשן עצים לחות לחות רב. וגם עלי הצמחים יוריקו ויפלו וישרו בלא זמני נפילתם. והפירות יתעפשו במהרה. וגם הבעלי חיים יברחו ממקום חנייתם והעופות יברחו מקניהם. וזה שהבורא הטביע בעופות ובב"ח הרגשת האוירים ובחור באוירים הטובים ולברוח מהאוירים הרעים והמעופשים והנפסדים ובפרט קצת מיני העופות כעורב למינו וסוס עגור. וכאשר יראו האותות האלה כולם או קצתם יוכל להקדים הרופ' הידיעה שהקדחות תהיינה דבריות. ואולם בעלי משפטי הכוכבים

[138א]

ידעו זה מצד משפטי הכוכבים וחבוריהם והלקויות ומשפטי העתים כמו שהוא מבואר בחכמה ההיא. וזה אין לרופא מצד שוא בעל מלאכת הרפואה לדעת זה לפי שחכמת הרפואה לא לעבור הדברי' המקובלי' מבעלי חכמת הטבע והדברי' הידועים בחכמת הרפואה. מפרק

כשיהיה עם קדחת שלשול ממין דבר שנתך ונמס הנה אותה הקדחת היא דבריית כי זה מקרה שאינו נפרד מהקדחות הדבריות

פרק בקדחות הדבריות הלחיות

פרק בקדחות הדבריות הלחיות כבר אמרנו שעפוש הרוח כאשר יתעבר הפסדו לליחות ויתלקח בהם ואם יתחדש מהרה מאחת או משתים או יותר קדחות תהיינה אותותיהם מן קדחת אחרת בלתי דברית שתהיינה מכיוצא בליחה ההיא וזה מצד היותה לחיית ויחזקו קצת המקרים מצד דבריותיה . ויעזור הרופא כשיהיה לחיית דבריית באותות המשיגות ומקדימות יעזרו יותר לידיעת זה ויהיו השתן והדפק ושאר האותות והמקרים באותות ומהם קדחת ליחיית כזאת שנכתבו בספרי החכמים מן הרופאים. ולפי שישתתף עם אותותיהם הליחיות קצת אותות קדחת דבריית כמו שאמרנו והיא רב המצוקה לעפוש הרוח ונפילת הכח ההוים [[ההוים]] בקדחות לסבה מבוארת אינם סגולה לקדחת הדבריית שהמקרים האלה נמשכים לכל עפוש רוח בגויה מאיזה צד שיהיה אבל הם מקרה לחום נכרי [שוה רוח] שוה יהיה זה השנוי לעפוש הרוח כמו בקדחות הדבריות ~~האמיתית~~ או בקדחת הדבריית הלחיית שנתעפש בה הרוח ראשונה ושנית הליחה או שיהיה זה לעפוש רוח הלב בסבת שכונת ליחה מעופשת שנתעפשה ראשונה ונתחלק שנית העפוש ברוח כמו שהוא בדלקת ובקדחות הלבניות והאדומיות הליחיות בלתי דבריות או להפעליות נפשיות ככעס והיגון והפעליות אחרות משנים מזג הרוח. **ואמנם** רוב המצוקה בקדחות ומהירות נפילת הכח לא בסבה מבוא[ר]ת הנה סגול[ה] בקדחת הדבר.

ולא מהתפשטות הקדחות

[118ב]

הרעות במקומות רבים ילקח ראיה על היותם דבריות כי אין התפשטות לחליים למזונות שנוי אנשי המקום מנהגם מזונות שלא היו רגילים בהם או זולתם מן הסבות באיכות חמים או קרים לחים או יבשים נתחדשו באויר מאיכות בלתי מעופש ולשנוי מזגו היו קדחות ליחיות או חלאים אחרים בכלל הגויה או באבר המיוחד. כשנתפשט הרמד או השעול במחוז מה לשנוי מזג הליחות יקולקל ערכיהם והוכנו לקבול חלאים מה ולא יקרה חולי דבריי ואויר דבריי אלא אותם שנשתנו לחום ולחות מעופש באיכות ארסיי אך ראוי שתדע שהמצוקות הלחיות הבלתי דבריות לשאיפת[13] האויר המעופש שהוא סבה מיוחדת ותמידית בהנה.

פרק בהנהגת האנשים בדבר והנהגת הקדחות הדבריות האמתיות המזוקקות הנהגת הקדחות והנהגת הקדחות הדבריות והן אותם שקרו לעפוש אויר והפסדו הפסד ועפוש הרוח אשר בלב לא הליחות כאשר יודע לך שהאויר דברי

ושהקדחות[14] דבריות מאותותיהן אשר אמרנו שים השגחתך לתקן האויר והנהגת האנשים בדברים המסירים העפוש. וזה שתסיר השכונות המעופשות ומפסידות האויר אם היו הדברי' [ה]מעופשים[15] אחד מהדברים הארציים שאמרנו בסבות ושתתקן האויר

---

13. בכת"י "לשאוית".

14. בכת"י "בהקדמקמות".

15. בכת"י "כמעופשים".

כבר אמרנו שעפוש הרוח כאשר יתמיד יתעבר הפסדו לליחות ויתלקח בהם. ואם יתחדש מהנה מאחת או משתים או יותר קדחות תהיינה אותותיהם כאותות קדחת אחרת בלתי דבריית שתתהוה מכיוצא בליחה וזה מצד היותה לחיית ויחזקו קצת המקרים מצד דבריותה. ויעזור הרופ' כשהיא לחיית דבריית באותות המשיגות ובמקדימות יעזור אותם לידיעת זה. ויהיו האותות מהשתן והדפק ושאר המקרים כאותות מקרה קדחת לחיית כמו שנכתבו בספרי חכמי הרופאים. ולא שיצטרך עם אותותיהם הלחיו' קצת איכות קדחות דבריות כמו שאמרנו והוא רוב המצוקה לעפוש הרוח ונפילת הכחות מהרה וזולת אלה שהמצוקה אינה מופלגת ונפילת הכחות ההווים בקדחות לסבה מבוארת אינה סגולה לקדחת דבריית שהמקרים כאלה נמשכים לכל עפוש רוח בגוויה מאי זה צד שיהיה אבל הם מקרה לחום נכרי מגיע

[138ב]

ללב שוה מזג כחו שוה יהיה זה השינוי לעפוש הרוח לבד כמו בקדחת דבריית האמתיית או בקדחת שנתעפש הרוח ראשונה ושנית הליחה או שיהיה זה סבה לעפוש רוב[3] הלב בסבת שכונת ליחה מעופשת שנתעפשה ראשונה ונתלקח שנית העפוש ברוח כמו שהוא בקדחו' הלבניות והאדומיות הלחיות בלתי דבריות. או להתפעלות נפשיות כמו כעס ויגון ואנחה והתפעליות אחרים משנים מזה הרוח, ואמנם רב המצוקה בקדחות ומהירות נפילת הכח ללא סבה מבוארת הוא סגולה בקדחת הדבר.

ולא מהתפשטות הקדח'

הרעות[4] במקומות רבים ילקח ראיה על היותם דבריות כי אין ההתפשטו' בחליים סגולה בדבריות כי ההתפשטות יהיה בכל החליים למזונות שינוי המקום

ומנהג אנשיה במזונות שלא היו רגילים בהם או זולתם מהסבות באיכיות בלתי מעופש. ולשינוי מזגם יהיו הקדחות לחיות או חליים אחרים בכלל הגוויה או באבר מיוחד. בשנה אחת יתפשט הר"מד או השעול במחוז מה לשינוי מזג הליחות וקלקול ערכיהם והוכנו לקבול חליים מה לא יקראו חולי דבריי ואויר דבריי אלא אותם שישתנו לחום ולחות מעופש באיכות ארסיי. אך ראוי שתדע שהמצוקות ונפילת הכח בתחלת החולי בעצם הקדחות הדבריות יותר מתמידים וחזקים ממה שיהיה בקדחות לחיות בשאיפת האויר המעופש שהוא סבה מיוחדת ותמידית בהנה.

פרק *בהנהגת האנשים בדבר והנהגת הקדחו' הדבריות המזוקקות*

הנהגת הקדחו' הדבריות וכן אותן שקרו לעפוש אויר והפסדו הפסד עפוש הרוח אשר בלב לא הליחות. כאשר יודע לך שהאויר מעופש

[139א]

3 לתקן לקרוא "רוח" במקום "רוב".

4 "הרעות" – המעתיק תקן בשוליים.

שנתעפש בעשונים והזניות מדברים קרים ויבשים מבושמי' הריח וקצת מן הסמים[16] הסגוליים בהסרת העפוש המאייכים האויר באיכות בלתי מקבל העפוש עד שהסבה המעופשת הארציית מן השכונות המפסידות[17] לא תעשינה רושם באויר. וגם אם היו הסבות שמימיות תמנענה ההכנות האלה האויר מקבל רושם בעת שפע הכוכב ששפע הכוכב הרע יעשה רושם באיש ובמקום המוכנים לטבעם לקבל השפע ההוא

[119א]

[[ההוא]]. ולא יעשה רושם בבלתי מוכנים לקבל זה. והם אותם שמזגם חולק והפכי לזה השפע. ולולא זה כבר היו כל האנשים אשר עומדים באויר הדבריי יחלו חליים דברי[י]ם בעת הדבר ימותו מהם או יבראו ואיננו כן שיש שיחלו ויש שלא יחלו וסבת זה ההכנה לקבול השפע והבלתי הכנה. ולכן היה תקון האויר בדברים מאיכים האויר באיכות חלוקה לעפוש מן הדברים היותר טובים שיעשו לאויר הדבריי בהנהגת הבריאות לרפואת הקדחות [[הקדחות]] האלו וכן הנהיג האנשים בהנהגת מזונות וריחות תכיננה הליחות והרוחות להיות ח[ו]לקות והפכיות לעפוש עד שימנע או שימעט קבולם רושם מאויר המפסיד. וזה כשישרפו עצים וירבו המוקדים במקום הדבריי וכ"ש מעצים רחניים עצי הדס ועשבי[18] האיזוב ורימוני[19] גיונברי ואתרוג ושאר מן האילנות המבושמות החולקים לעפוש בבשמיות עשונם

ואשר יכלה העפוש מן האויר. ויריחו האנשים מאלה טבולים בחומץ ומעלה האתרוג ועשבי[20] נמאס הנקרא שרפול ויזו המקומות במים וחומץ ששרה בהם צנדליש כתוש ורדים והדס מ"א עשה חלקים לבונה חלק עלי אתרוג ועלי נמאס עלי אזוב מ"א שני חלקים ויוזה מהם המקום באויר הדבריי

ויבואו במקומות האבניים ובספים[21] ובבתים הרצופים באבנים תחתיים מוזים בזה שקדם זכרו, וכ"ש בעת השינה שהכחות נרדמים ולא יחלקו על האיכיות הרעות הנשאפות כמו שיחלקו בעת התעוררם והיותם זריזות ובפועל. ולזאת הסבה תמנע השינה לנוש כי[22] הארסיים ולבעלי המורסות הארסיות ולמחנקים ובהתחלת עונות הקדחת. ויהיו המזונות מן התרנגולים והתרנגולות והגדים והעגל[י]ם והעופות הארציים המדבריים הקטנים במינם צלויים באש או במרק או בחומץ ועסיס רמונים ובוסר ומיץ לימוניש וחמוץ האתרוג ולא בכבשים וירחקו החזיר אוכליו וישמרו מן הקרבים

---

16 בכת"י "החמים," ותיקנתי לפי פאריש.

17 בכת"י "המסידות".

18 בכת"י "עצבי".

19 בכת"י "רומני".

20 בכת"י "עשני".

21 בפאריש "בספים," גירסה יותר הגיונית מה"ברפים" בליידן .

22 כנראה המעתיק היה מבולבל. השווה פאריש בו נמצא "לנשוכי," נוסח מובן.

ושהקדחות דבריות לאותותיהם אשר אמרנו שים השגחתך לתקן האויר והנהגת האנשים בדברים מסירים העפוש. וזה שתסור מהשכונות המעופשות המפסידות האויר אם ~~באו~~ היו[5] הדברים המעפשים אחד מהדבריי' ארציים שאמרנו בסבות. ושתתקן האויר המעופש בעשונים וזלופים מדברים קרים ויבשים ומבשמי' הריח' וקצת מהסמים הסגוליים בהסרת העפוש [~~ומא~~] המאייכים האויר באיכות בלתי מקבל העפוש עד שהסבה המעופשת הארציית לא יעשה רושם באויר וגם אם היו הסבות שמימיות תמנעם ההקטרות האלה. דע שהאויר מקבל רושם בעת שפע הכוכב עד שהכוכב הרע יעשה רושם באישי המקום המוכנים בטבעם לקבול זה

והם אותם שמזגם חלק הפכיי לזה השפע. ולולי זה כבר היו כל האנשים אשר באויר הדברי מתפעלים ויחלו חליים דבריים וימותו מהם או יבריאו ואיננו כן כי יש שיחלו ויש שלא יחלו. וסבת זה ההכנה לקבול השפע והבלתי הכנה. ולכן היה תקון האויר בדברי' מאייכים האויר איכות חולקת לעפוש. ומן הדברי' היותר טובים שיעשו לאויר המעופש הדבריי בהנהגת הבריאות ולרפ[ו]את הקדחות האלה להנהיג האנשי' בהנהגת המזונות וריחות תכוננה קטורם רושם הליחות והרוחות להיותם חולקות והפכיות לעפוש עד שימנע או ימעט קבולם רושם האויר המפסיד וזה כשישרפו עצים ריחניים וירבו המוקדים במקו' הדבריי' וכ"ש בעצי הדס ורוש מרין וערער ואתרוג ועשב אזוב ושאר מהאילנות והעשבים המבושמי' החולקים לעפוש בבשמיות עשונם

[139ב]

ואשר יכלה עפוש האויר הוא שיריחו האנשים בגדים טבולים בחומץ ויריחו עלי האתרוג וצירפוייל. ויזלפו המקומות במים וחומץ ששרה בתוכם צנדלי כתושים ורדים והדס מכל אחד י' חלק' לבונה חלק. עלי אתרוג עלי שירפוייל אנ" שני חלקים ויוזה מזה המקום אשר יעמדו בו ויושטחו יריעות בחלונות טבולות במים האלה וינעלו השערים. ויסתר האדים ממקום גבוה באויר הדבריי ויבואו במקומות האבניים ובספים ובבתים הרצופים באבנים מזולפים בזה. וכ"ש בעת השינה שאז הכחות נרדמים ולא יחלקו אל האיכויות הרעות הנשאפות כמו שיחלקו בעת התעוררותם. ולזאת הסבה תמנעו השינה לנשוכי הארסיים ולבעלי המורסות הארסיות וגם למחנקים ולהתחלת עונות הקדחות. ויהיו מזונותיהם מן התרנגולים והתרנגולות והגדיים והעגלים היונקים והעופות הארציים והמדבריים הקטנים במינם צלויים באש או במרק וחומץ ועסיס רימונים ובוצר ומיץ לימונש וחומצת אתרוג. ולא ירבו באכילת הכבשים ~~וירו~~ וירחיקו החזיר אוכליו וישמרו מהקרבים.

וגם ישמרו מאכילת הדגים אך מהסלעיי האדום המקושקש ודרך אכילתו לפעמים במרחשת עם חומץ ואזוב ומעט בצל ודרציני וישמרו מעופות המים ויהיו רוב התבלין שיאכלו צנדלי ודרציני. וישמרו מאכילת פירות המתוקים וכ"ש מהתאנים הלחים. ומהתפלים כמו קשואים ואבטיחים. ויוכלו לאכול כל פרי חמוץ קוהא קובץ ועפוץ כמו רימונים ותפוחים חמוצים בעלי הריח ממוצעים ופרונש שחורות ואגסים והחבושים

---

5 "אם היו" – תקון בשוליים.

[119ב]

וישמרו מן הדג אך מהסלעי האדום המקושקש

לפעמים במרחשת וחומץ ואזוב ומעט בצל ודרציני. וישמר מעופות המים ויהיו רוב תבליניו הדרציני הטוב והסובל. וישמר מאכילת הפירות המתוקי' וכ"ש מתאנים ומהתפלים בקשואים ואבטיח. יוכל לאכול פרי חמוץ קוהה קובץ ועפץ כרמונים ותפוחים ריחנים מבושמים ממוצעים ופרונש שחורות פיראש וחבושים

ואפרסקים טבולים ביין ישתה היין הריחני מזוג ויריחנו וישמר מן הגבנה ומן החלב ויאכל מעט מן הבצל בחומץ בתחלת מאכלו וישתו האנשים בכל בקר יין משובח לבן ויאכלנו אחריו ממרקחת הלימוניש במשקל חצי אשקריפול שהוא עשרה גרעיני חטה טיט חתום או מזה המשקה. יוקח קלפת האתרוג אפסנתין רענן גניי אזוב הדס מ"א אוקי' טיט ארמיני וטיט חתום מ"א דרהם סוכרי ג' ליטרים מי ורד חצי ליטר ויעשה מש[ק]ה והוא מסיר העפושים מחזק הכחות מאד ויזהיר הרוחות ויבשלו במשקה אחר הזדככו בדלחים צחים[23] מאובקים ב' דר' אודם ג' הם גראנט בהירים מאובקי' צרורים בבגד משי לבן או תולעת שני ויהיו תמיד בכלי משמרת המשקה. וישמר האדם מן הריחות הנפסדים מאד. **ויריקו האנשים** מותרי ליחותיהם אם יגבר בכח הדם יוקזו[24] ואם תגבר אחת הליחות יחקנה כראוי מפחד שתלקה האויר בליחות המותריות והרוחות מ[ה]רה ללחות הנובע[25] בסבתם מנגד לעפושים תפוח להריח מצנדלים שלשתם קנמון בשם מכ"א דר' לבונה חצי אוק' כפרים מור מאה גרעינים ארבאטור ג' דרה' דרציני ב' דר' ירוקו גם מזה עשה מוגמר בלילה בעת הבית סגור. ויוזה בעת ההקטרה ממי ההזיה הנזכרת למעלה.

פרק בהנהגת המוקדחי' בקדחת הדבר המזוקקת העתיקהו מן האויר ההוא אם

[120א]

אם אפשר ואם לא תקן על הדרך הנזכר בפרק שלפני זה ופנה לחזק הלב במזון ובדברים רפואיים גם בתרנגולים הצלויים בדברים חמוצים ומרק העדשים והמאכלים הלבנים במיץ לימוניש וימעטו בהם השקדים והקמחים. וישתו היין הלבן הריחני הקהה מעט ועסיס הרמונים וחמוץ אתרוג ששרה בו טיט חתום וטיט ארמיני ויאכל הפירות החמוצים ובפרט הרמונים והתפוחים המתוקים הממוצעים והפירניש שנתבשלו באילנם וגדגדאניות[26] קוהות וחזרת בחומץ. ויאכל מאכל מיץ ורדים ומרקחת מיץ לימוניש ויריח הצנדליש ההיכל וההדס ומי הורדים שישרה כפר וזעפראן מ"א משקל גרעיני חטה. לבונה חצי דרהם קנמון בושם דרהם. הדס רענן כתוש אוקי' מי ורד ליטר' ורתח רתיחה ויושמו בכלי כסף או זכוכית אם אי אפשר בכסף ויוטבלו בם בגדי משי לבן ויונח בפנים והאף והידיים ויעשו[27] על הלב הנחות מבגדי משי לבן או תולעת שני טבולים במי ורדים הנזכרים ומעט טין ומיץ תפוחים ומעט חומץ. ומעט השינה.

---

23 בכת"י "צחיק".

24 בכת"י כתוב "יוזקו".

25 בכת"י "הטבע" אמנם צריך להיות "הנובע" כמו בפאריס.

26 שם לועזי בשביל מירובילנס. ראה הערתי לתרגום.

27 אולי "וינוחו?"

[140א]

והאפרסקים טבולים ביין וישתו יין ריחני מזוג כראוי, וישמרו עצמם מחלב וגבינה. ויאכלו מעטי בצל עם חומץ בתחלת המאכל, וישתו האנש' בכל בקר יין לבן משובח ויאכלו אחריו ממרקחת הלימו' במשקל חצי ℈[6] שהוא עשרה גרעיני חטה עם טיט חתום. או ישתו מזה המשקה: **סם** קליפת אתרוג אפסנתין רענן גניי. אזוב הדס. אנ. ℥.[7] דרציני. צנדלי. אנ. חצי ℥ טין ארמיני. טיט חתום אנ. ʒ[8] סוכרי ג' ליטר. מי ורדים חצי ליטר' יעשה משקה והוא מסיר העפושים ומחזק הכחות מאד ויזהיר הרוחות. ויבשלו במשקה אחרי הזדככו בדולחים צחים מאובקים. ב' ʒ או גראנדש בהירים מאובקים צרורים בבגד משי או תולעת שני. ויהיו תמיד בכלי למשמרת . וישמרו מהריחות הנפסד' ויריקו האנשים מותרי ליחותם

אם יגבר בהם הדם יוקזו. או אם תגבר אחת מהליחות יורקו כראוי מפחד מהתלקח עפוש אויר בליחות המותריות והרוחות מהרה ללחות הנובע בסבתם מנגד העפושים.

תואר תפוח להריח. **סם** ג' מיני צנדליש. קנמון בושם מכל אחד ʒ לבונה חצי ℥' כפירים מור. אנ.ה. gf ג' ʒ דרציני. ב' ʒ . צנדלי מוקציליני משקל פשוט. בלהאן[9] ʒ. לפדנום. אנ. ט .ʒ. עלך אלבנוס ʒ ירוקה וגם מזה יעשה מוגמר יקוטר בלילה הבית סגור ויוזה בעת ההקטרה עם המים הנזכרי' למעלה

פרק

בהנהגת המוקדחים בקדחת האויר[10] המזוקקת

ההנהגה העתיקהו מן האויר ההוא אם אפשר ואם לאו תתקן האויר על הדרך

[140ב]

שזכרנו. ופנה לחזק הלב בכל עוז במזון ובדברים רפואיים. גם בתרנגולים הצלויים טבולים עם דברים חמוצים ומרק העדשים והמאכלים הלבנים עם מיץ לימונש וימעטו בהם שקדים וקמחים. וישתה היין הלבן הריחני קוהה מעט ועסיס רימונים וחמוץ האתרוג ששרה בו טין ארמיני וטיט חתום. ויאכל הפירות החמוצים ובפרט הרימונים והתפוחים הריחניים הממוצעים. והפרונש הלבנות שנתבשלו באילנם וצבעם כצבע אלבירגיניש קהות. ויאכל חזרת בחומץ וגם ממרקחת מיץ ורדים ומרקחת מיץ לימונש ויריח הצנדליש וההדס ומי ורדים שישרה בהם כופר וזערפן אנ. י' גרעינים. לבונה חצי ʒ. קנמון בושם. ʒ. הדס רענן כתוש ℥' מי ורדים. ℥' יורתח זה ויונח בכלי כסף או בכלי זכוכית יוטבלו בם בגדי משי לבן ויונח בפנים והידים והאף.

---

6 שקרופל.

7 אוקיה (או אונקיה).

8 דראכם.

9 או "כלהאן." אולי עשב שקראוהו כולאן הינדי, סוג של ליציאום?

10 צ"ל "הדבר" במקום "האויר".

ואין ראוי שתקרב להריק שום הרקה בתרופה משלשלת שלא תריק הרוח שהוא נתך ופורח בהרקה וכ"ש הקדחת הזאת ההו[א] ברוח ההלום במהלומות האויר הדבריי. ואין לתגבורת ליחה יחוייב להריקה ותורקנה הטובות הצריכות הגויה ויורק הרוח עמהם. ועוד שרוב המשלשלים יש בהם כארסיות ונגוד למזג הבר[י]א ולכחות הלב. ולא יקיז בשום פנים מצד הקדחת הזאת אלא אם יצטרך הקזה לצד אחר יוקז אחר השקול המאוזן. וכן אם צריך לחוקן כך מוצא עשה בשקול הדעת הצודק. וישתו המשקה הזה. יוקח אבוקדולה הוא חמצאעת ליטר' משינה אוק' צנדלים מי ורד ליטרא ואולש רעננות או יבשות מנוקות מיתדותיהם ועוקציהם רביע ליטרא עסיס רמונים שרויים יין מ"א רביע ליטר' מיץ הדס אוקי' וחצי

[120ב]

סוכרי ג' ליטר' עשה המשקה ישרו בו בדולחים צחים אודם בהיר מאובקים מ"א דר' צרורים בצרור משי שתה במים לפי הרצון הצאנדיל והויאוליש והחמצאניות והמשי ישרה כתוש יום ולילה ואחר יעשה המשקה.

פרק בהנהגת המוקדחים בקדחות דבריות לחיות דע כי אין הפרש בין הנהגת המוקדחים האלה ובין הנהגת המוקדחים משאר הקדחות העלפיות[28] או דמיות או אדומיות או לבניות פשוטות או מורכבות הדמיות יוקזו והאדומיות והלבניות ישולשלו בעליהן ותונהגנה הליחיות במזונות ותרופות עם שמירת תנאי הענינים בכל אחד תונהגנה הקדחות הדבריות הלחיות בהנהגת הקדחות הליחיות יחוייב שתהיה הפניה לחזק הלב יותר חזקה מן הבלתי דבריית וראוי שיפנה לזונו יותר ממה שיפנה לזון מוקדחים הבלתי דבריות במזונות נאותים לקדחת הלב. גם לפעמים בבלתי נאות לקדחת אלא שהוא יותר ערב ונכסף למוקדח ונהוג שהכחות מתחזקים. ויעשה זה בהשגחה ועיון מופלג להאכיל הבשר ולשתות היין הריחני רב המזג שהצורך לעיון בזאת יותר לצורך ההשגחה בליחה ורוח וכח. יעוין רופא בהנהגת מוקדחים הליחות וינהיגם[29] בהנהגתם פונה ומשגיח להנהגה הדבריית הנזכרת למעלה מתקון האויר. ועזבתי זכרון ההנהגה מזה המאמר[30] שלא היתה בכוונה בו ביאור הנהגתם ולכן תלקח ממאמריהם וביאורם שחיברו כל אחד מגדולי המלאכה הזאת.

פרק בקדחות שקרו בזאת השנה. המאמ' הזה חברתיו ביחוד לבאר בהנהגת הקדחות שקרו בשנה הזאת ומקריהן ואותותין המשיגים והמפורסמים גם להמון וכ"ש לחכם רופא ולפי האותות לא יספק אחד מן החכמים כשאינן דבריות אמתיות[31] שהוא תראינה באותות ומקרי הלחיית אלא אם יש ספק ישנו אם הם קדחות דבריות לחיות הנה לחות עלופיות לבד

[121א]

לבד להדמות אותותיהן המשיגים שהמצוקות והעלופים ירבו בליחות הדבריות ובליחות העלופיות בלתי דבריות. ומה שיבאר הספק הוא האותות המקודמות הלקוחות מתכונת האויר אם הוא דבריי אם לא ובסבות הדבריות אם קדמו. והנה לא נראו האותות באויר (באויר) באביב ולא בסתו ולא מערפליות ושאר ובריחת העופות מקניהן והרמשים

28. בכת"י "הלעפיות".

29. בכת"י "ויניהגם".

30. בכת"י "האמאמר".

31. מודגש בכת"י.

ויעשו על הלב הנחות מבגדי משי לבן או תולעת שני טבולים עם מי ורדים ומעט יין ומיץ תפוחים ומעט חומץ וימעיט השינה .

ואין ראוי ש[ת]קרב להריק שום הרקה וכ"ש בתרופה משלשלת שלא תריק הרוח הנתק ופורח בהרקה וכ"ש במהלומות האויר. ואין הקדחת הזאת ההוא לתגבורת הליחה יחוייב להריקה כי תורקנה הטובות הצריכות לגוייה ותורק הרוח עמהם. ועוד שרוב המשלשלים יש בהם ארסיות ונגוד למזג הבריא ולכחות הלב. ולא יוקז בשום פנים בקדחת הזאת ואם יצטרך להקזה יוקז מצד אחד אחר השקול המאוזן בעת. וכן אם יצטרך אל חוקן רק מוצא הפרש יעשהו עם שקול הדעת צודק וישתה המשקה הזה: סם

אסיטושא ליטר. משינא ʒ' צנדלי. מי ורדים

[141א]

אנ' חצי ליטר ויאולי לחות או יבשות מנוקות מעוקציהם רביע ליטר. עסיס רימונים רביע ליטר מיץ רימונים. ʒ'. מיץ עלי הדס ʒ' וחצי. סוקרי. ג'. ליטרי. יעשה מזה משקה ישרו בו בדולחים צחים ואודם בהיר מאובקים צרורים בצרור בגד משי. אנ'. י' גרעינים ישתה מזה לפי הרצון. הצנדלי והויאו' והאסטושא ישרו כתושים יום ולילה אחת תוך המיצים הנזכרים ואחר כן יעשה משקה.

פרק *בהנהגת המוקדחים מקדחו' דבריות ליחיות*

דע כי אין הפרש בהנהגת המוקדחים משאר הקדחות העלופיות הלחיות הדמיות אדומיות או לבניות פשוטות או מורכבות אלא שהדמיות יוקזו. והאדומיות והלבניות ישולשלו בעליהן. ותונהגנה הלחיות במזונות ותרופות עם שמירת תנאי הענינים בכל אחת ואחת. תונהגנה הקדחו' הדבריות הלחיות בהנהגת הלחיות בלתי דבריות. אלא שבקדחות הדבריות הלחיות יחוייב שתהיה ההשגחה לחזק הלב יותר חזקה מהבלתי דבריות. וראוי שיפנה לזונו יותר ממה שיפנה לזון מוקדחי הבלתי דבריות במזונות נאותים לקדחת וללב. גם לפעמים בבלתי נאותים לק[ד]חת אלא שהוא יותר ערב ונכסף למוקדח. וכבר ידענו שהכחות מתחזקים בערב אמנם יעשה זה בהשגחה ועיון מופלג. וראוי להאכילו הבשר הנאות לו וישקהו היין הריחני רב המזג שהצורך לעיון בזה יותר ראוי בהשגחה ממה שראוי בליחה ולרוח ולכח. יעיין הרופא בהנהגת מוקדחי הליחות וינהיגם בהנהגתם פונה ומשגיח להנהגת הדבריות הנזכרות למעלה מתקון האויר. ***תם ונשלם תהלה לאל עולם.***

[The Paris text concludes here.]

מחוריהן. ולא נראה בפירות[32] עפוש יותר מן העפוש הרגיל הטבעי[33] להם. ואיך שיהיה הנה לחיים עלופיים שוה יהיה לחיים דבריים או לבד לחיים. וראוי שינהגו בהקזה או בהרקה אחרת לפי תגבורת הליחות המעופשות וכאשר עיינתי בהם באישים רבים הן לחיות מעורבבות לא פשוטות ותגבורת דם ומימיות רבי האויריות רבי הכמות כאלו הם לחות ארסיות לרוב עפושם והפסדם לרוב כמותם ודע איכותם תתעוררנה בתחילה המנצחות לטבע ולכן יתעורר הטבע כנגדם בתחלתן לדחות הליחה והחומר המימיי בזיעה וזיעות מעלפות. כי כשתהיינה קצתו עב לא ינקה בזיעה ולא בהתחלה אך ירתח בהתעוררות החומר להתנער בזיעה ויציק החומר העב ההוא בהרתחת ולא יתנקה. ואם קרה שיתנקה בשלשול או קיא או רעפית דם חזקים או בשאר עתות החולי או מעצמו או במלאכה רפואיית אולי ירפאו. ונראה ברבים בשנה הזאת שקרה להם שלשול או קיא או רעיפת דם נחירים חזקים ורבים נרפאו ועמד כחם והיו מהם שימותו מנפילת כח ברוב ההרקה ופתאומיות ואע"פ שהיתה ראויה לפי החומר ורבויו כמו שימותו בעלי היציאות רבות המוגלא ובעלי השקוי אם תורק מהם המוגלא או המים בבת אחת להמשך הרוח הנושא לכחות ופרחו על הליחה המורקת.

ואפשר שהיתה סבת הקדחות האלה חמריות ר"ל מרוע הנהגת המזונות בכמותם ואיכותם כי היתה יוקר ומעט

[121ב]

המצא[34] מזונות הנאכלים הנהוגים בחמשת מיני התבואה ואכלו רוב העם לחם גרגרים וזרעים בלתי נהוגים חרצון וערמון ואלונים נראה שהיתה הסבה שמימיית בקדחות השנה איך האויר והליחות איכות בלתי דבריי וחדש בליחות כלנה רוע איכות ואמת כי היה שנדבקו מאדים והשמש במעלה הראשונה מטלה ומאדים הוא כוכב שברצון האל מרבה החום והשרפה [[והשרפכה]] והרתיחה באויר והלחות והשמש מעורר חום ומרבהו והמזל והמעלה שנדבקו שם הוא מעלה ומזל פני מאדים וממשלתו כשהוא שם רבה ועצומה להעיר ביסודות והנמזגים מהם מה שנבראו להעיר והוא החום והרתיחה והשריפה והיה זה ביום בא השמש בטלה שהוא השווי האביבי שיש אי זה כוכב שיהיה לו ממשלת ביום ההוא ממשלה נצבת כל השנה וכ"ש בזמן הקיץ. וטלה ששם היה הדבוק מורה על חליי המוח ומפני שהיה החום והרתיחה הוא הגובר בסבת זה הדבוק התחייב לפיהו ברצון האל עליית החליים למוח כברסם ושאר החליים רתיחת הליחות בגדרי והחצבה וברצון האל נותן ממשלה והשפעה לכוכבים ולמקומות השמים על הארץ ויתחדשו איכיות בתחתונים ביסודות ובמזגים מהם התחדשו בעולם החליים והקדחות האלה במקומות והאישים המוכנים לקבלם לאשר הביא האל י"ת וי"ת ואע"פ שאין העיון לסבה השמימיית והסגוליית[35] לרופא מצד שהוא רופא אך מצד שהוא אצטגניניי או אלהיי ובעל תורה ראיתי להזכיר הסבה הזאת הנה מפני שהתפארו קצת המתחכמי' לאמר שהחליים דבריים מפני שחייבם הדבוק. ואמנם שהם היו מן החליים המתפשטים ואולם עזר בהולדם הדבוק אך לא כל חולי מתפשט ואשר יחייבהו הדבוק או ממשלת כוכב דבריי וגם לא התחייב לפי משפטי הכוכבים שימשך לדבוק הזה תולדת איכות דבריי אמתי אשר גדרנוהו אך התחייב אם רצה האל רתיחת

[122א]

---

32 בכת"י "בפירוש".

33 בכת"י "הטבע".

34 בכת"י "הצמא".

35 בכת"י "והמגוליית".

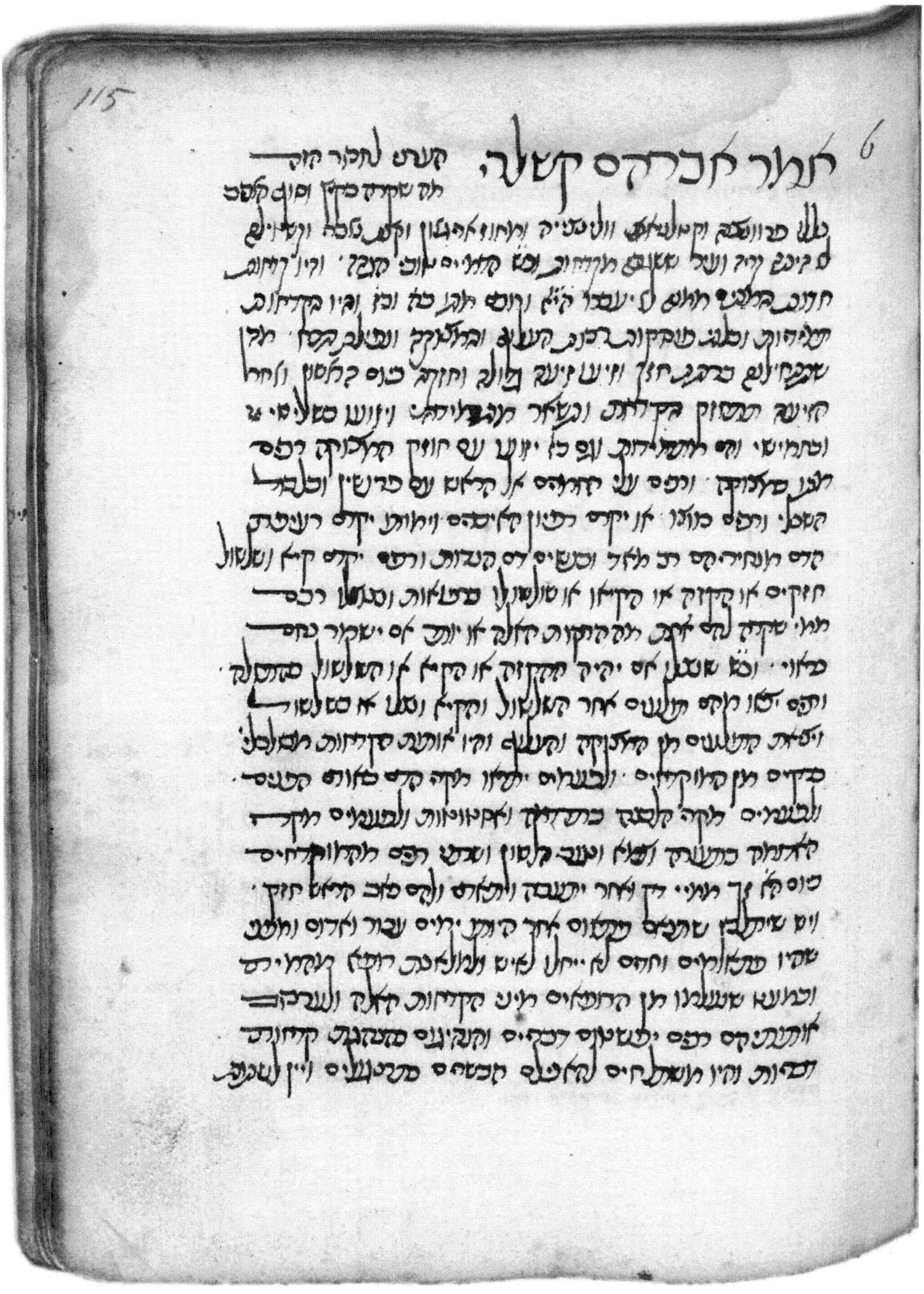

Figure 4. The opening page of Abraham's plague tractate in one of the two surviving manuscript copies, produced about a century after the tractate's composition. The untitled folio is from Leiden, Leiden University Library, MS or. 4778, fol. 115a. Reproduced courtesy of Leiden University Library.

הליחות ושריפתן ועליית החליים באברים העליונים.

ההנהגה בקדחות שקרו באלה שכלנה ממין [[אחד]] אחד ובמקרים דומים מתחלפים בכחות והיותר ראוי בהתחלה שיותר בטנם ויוצא הפרש אם בחוקנים ואכילת המזונות הרפואיים המרויחים בירקות המרויחות שיש בהם קצת משלשל כסלקא ומרקיליאול וקושיש ומעט לבלב שלוקים במים ומעט *שמן ויאולט כבושים בחומץ עסיס רמונים ובוסר ענבים ישתה ממרקם והירקות תאכלנה. ואם*[36] ירויחו טוב ואם לא יורוח בזה יותן בערב השני חוקן ומן היותר טוב החוקן ביום הראשון והב' והג'. יוקז מוריד אמצעי או מורידי הראש מזרע ימין ושמאל כפי אשר ישוער הרופא יותר טוב ותהיה הקזה ביינונית בכמות לפי האיש והרגלו וכחו ומזגו ואם הוא נער ישרט אחורי האזנים ואם ירבה כאב ראשם עם כל השלשול או ההקזה תהיה ההקזה מן הצפון טובה וביום הד' ישולשלו במשלשל יהיה בו ויאולש פרונש תמר אינדי מנא נאר אנדי שנבר וריבברבר כולם או קצתם משיעור שיראה לרופא. ואם יראה שיושם פוליפודי יושם שזה המשלשל כולל הליחות כלנה שכלנה מעורבבות בחלאים האלה והוא קל בלתי חומץ כל הכחות שאין בו סם משלשל בעל איכות רעה ולא ארסיית. בקר וערב ירחצו שוקיהם ורגליהם בבשול עלי ערבה וגפנים ובאבונג בחפיפה רבה. ואם עם כל זה יכאב ראשם ויראו אותות עליית החולי אל הראש וכבר עברו הה' והז' ודקדקו ההנהגה ואולי חלשו הכח בסבול ההקזה כוללת תשולחנה העלוקות במצח והחוטם ויוקזו מורידי תחת הלשון. או ירעפו נחיריו וגלח ראשם וירחץ בבשול הדברים הנפים המקררים במעט הרתיעה יאוזנו לפי שקול דעת הרופא. ורדים ג' אוקיות כרכום אוקיא וחצי באבונג מלילוט מ"א אוקי' זה נאות

[122ב]

בתחלת עליית החולי מרתיע האדים העולים. מתיך האדים העשניים שעלו מבשל מישן משקיט הכאב. זה יעשה אחר חקוקן אך אם יהיה הכאב חזק במיץ חזרת ומיץ ורדים שוה בשוה חומץ אחד מעשרים ואם תרבה התעורה עם כל זה יחובש מצחם אחרי הרחיצה בזה. משיחה ורדיית פופוליאון מ"א אוק' שמן יברוח חצי אוק' שמן באבונג אוק' וחצי שעוה אוק' אם זעפראן מ"א חצי דרהם שעוה לבנה אוק' יעשה משיחה. ויזונו בשתיתות המבשלות בחלב זרע מלונש וימעיטו בחלב השקדים וכ"ש מהישני' שהם חמים מוסיפים בעצם המוח מכאיבות אותו. או יזונו במרק העדשים או מרק זרעונים ~~במעט מרק העדשים או הזרעונים~~ במעט פוטר[37] וחומץ ותבשיל הדלועים והירק הנזכר למעלה ולא תושמנה הבוראגיש בתבשיליהם. והפרוניש והתפוחים הריחניים והחזרת והרמון והלגלוגית[38] יופלו בהן. יתוקן אוירים תמיד בכזית בשול הדס וגפנים ועלי גפנים וקנים ודבר מועט מעלי אתרוג. ויסגרו החולנות המזרחיים והדרומיים תמיד ויורחצו זרועיהם וידיהם במים חמים שזה מועיל מאד מן המצוקה בלב מאיזה צד שיהיה ואחר הרחיצה בחמים תנוגבנה ותושמנה הידים לבד במים קרים ויעוררו מים חמים בתירוש תותים ומעט חומץ ומי ורד ויונח על לבבהן תמיד עלים גפנים טבולים בזה מי ורד חצי ליטר' יין לבן אוק' חומץ אוק' זעפראן משקל חצי פשוט. כפר משקל גרעין חטה צנדיל הכל חצי דר' בשול הדס ב' אונקיו' יעורב. ודע כי ראוי שישמרו מן הבשר והיין מאד אלא בהכרח פחד נפילת הכח המתחזק באכילת המזון המורגל המאוה יותר ממה שיתחזק בדברים ומזון הרפואי בלתי מורגלים ובלתי מאוים.

---

36 הקטע בין הכוכבים נשמט אצל פינקהוף.

37 יותר טוב: פיטר (פטרוסילה).

38 אולי "חלוגלוגות", שמשמעות "חלילג" באבן וואפיד היא מיראבולנש. ראה את ההערה בתרגום.

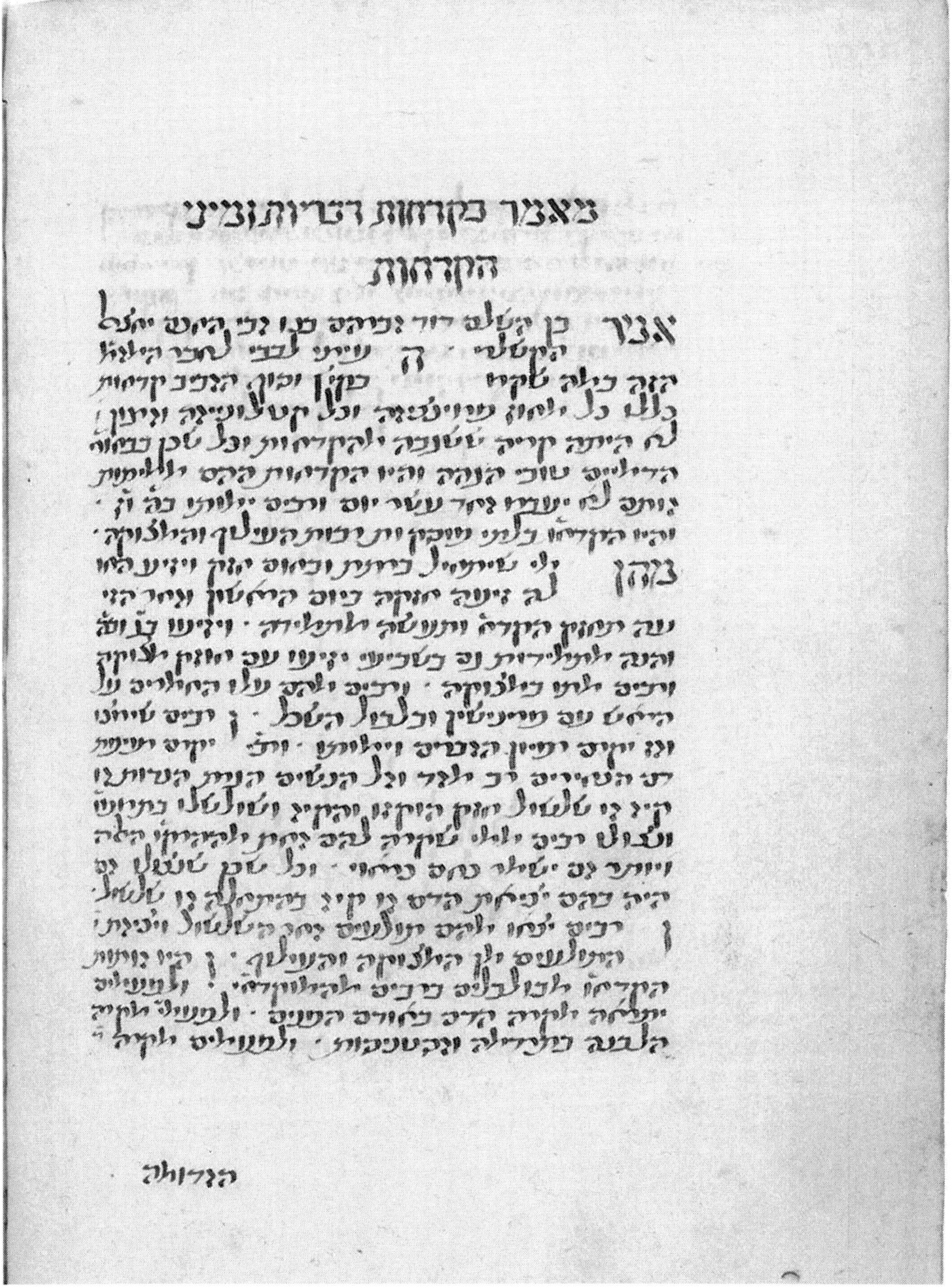
מאמר בקדחות דבריות ומיני
הקדחות

Figure 5. The opening page of Abraham's plague tractate in the second of the two surviving manuscript copies, produced about a century after the tractate's composition. Paris, BnF, MS héb. 1191, fol. 134b. Reproduced courtesy of the BnF.

משקה ישתו ממנו בקר וערב והוא מזון רפואיי מרווח מחזק הלב

[123א]

ממית ומוציא התולעים שרבו בחליים בשנה הזאת ומתקין הליחות מכינם להכין בשלשול ושתן וזיע. חמצאניות לפאס האגודה קפילי וניריש שורש שומר פוטר[39] שורש אשפרגי מ"א רביע ליטרא קלפת שורש תותים חצי ליטרא קלפת אפסנתין קלפת האתרוג הדס סומאק מ"א חצי אוק' פום טירא אוק' מיץ הנדבי מיץ לבלב מ"א ליטר מיץ קרישוש מיץ מרקואיל מ"א חצי ליטר' ויאוליש רביע ליטר מיץ ורדים משומרי' בסוכרי מיץ לימוניש דיאמינטא מ"א ב' אונקיות חומץ חצי אונק' עסיס רמונים חמוצים אוק' לכל ליטר' סוכרי ליטרא יבושל בשלמות ואם יהיה החולה מרווח יוסרו מיץ הלבלב והקרישש והמרקוריאל. וישים תמורת מיץ ורדים מי ורדים וישרה במשקה צנדיל אדום חצי אונק' סוס? ג' דר' ישתה בבקר אוק' וחצי לגדולים בד' אוק' וחצי מים חמים בשל בהם זרעונים מצטיק. ולקטני' שני כפות בעשרה ימים[40] שבשל בהם מעט מצטיק או סומאק.

ובמשיחה הצוריית יומשח בטנם או בזאת אם לא תוכן הצוריית: שמן אפסנתין. שמן שקדים מרים. בשול חצי אוק' סומאק. וחצי אוק' קלפת האתרוג ודרהם סינטוניקא חומץ עסיס רמונים מ"א ג' אונק' בשל יחד עד שישוב לשעור השמן. שעוה לבנה אוק' צבר חצי דר' יעשה משיחה.

משיחה וורדיית מי או מיץ ורדים חצי ליטר' מיץ פאפאויר מ"א רביע ליטר' ואם לא ימצא מיץ יושם תמורתו בשול זרע פאפאויר בשני ליטר' מים עד שישוב לחצי ליטר'. שמן זרעים שמן זרע דלועים ליטר' שמן באבונג רביע ליטר'. יבושל השמן במה שנזכר עד השאר השמן לבד על האש גחלים אז תותך שעוה לבנה ג' אוקיות ויוסר מעל האש עד שיקרש ויושם שם אבק זעפראן אבק אופי משקל פשוט.

משיחה צוריית לנו לארסיים

[123ב]

ולנחשים ותולעי הבטן ושאר איברי הגוף. יוקח מיץ סנטוריאה גדולה וקטנה. מיץ אפסנתין עלה אפרסק מ"א ליטר' מיץ לגלוגות[41] מיץ קרישפיניל חומץ עסיס רמונים מיץ לימוניש מ"א ליטר' יעורב ויובש ויודק החצי ויעורב בשמן ויעשה שמן. קמח לופינש ליט' סינאמומי לבונה מירא מ"א אוק' צבר צרי מ"א חצי אוק' מררת פר אוק' קלפת שורש תות ורמון. סומק גרעיני אתרוג מנוקים קלפת שורש פלגירה סינטוניקא זרע אלישנדרי זרע כרוב רודה מ"א חצי אונק' קלפת אתרוג יבשה דקה ג' אוק' טין חתום קרן צבי שרוף אוק' ויעורב עם אבק המיצים ויולש בהם הצבר והצרי והמירא יאבק היטב הראוי להאבק. וילקח שמן שקדים מרים שמן אפרסקים מ"א ד' ליטר' שמן ורד שמן מצטיק שמן נרדין מ"א ג' אונק' שעוה חצי ליטר' ויקפא ויעורב במשיחה האבק הנזכר היטב.

תם ונשלם תהלה לאל עולם

---

39 כנראה, "פיטר".

40 אולי מתכוון ל"מים"?

41 חלגלוגות?

TRANSLATION OF LEIDEN, LEIDEN UNIVERSITY LIBRARY, MS or. 4778, fols. 115a–123b[1]

ABRAHAM B. DAVID CASLARI: UNTITLED.

NLI, IMHM F 17378

[**fol. 115a**] [**Pinkhof 51**] Said Abraham Caslari: I was moved to [write] this composition by what happened in the summer and late spring across Provence, Catalonia, Valencia, the region of Aragon and parts of Navarre and Castile—**not a city or town was spared**[2] by the fevers. The fevers were acute and those who died of them did not last eleven days; most of them died on the first and seventh,[3] especially those who were sanguine and of good regimen. They were continuous fevers without intermittence, with much fainting, anguish, and loss of strength. Some of them commenced with strong shivering and sweating greatly on the first day, after which the fever strengthened and remained continuous. They sweated on the third and fifth [days], and they[4] were continuous; on the seventh, they also sweated with great anguish—many of them died in anguish. For many, the matter rose to the head, accompanied by phrenitis[5] and mental confusion.[6] Many weakened or experienced weakness in the limbs then died. They had great nose bleeds, or vaginal bleeding in women; many experienced strong vomiting and diarrhea. If they were treated with bloodletting, [induced] vomiting and purges, most of those who received one or more of these evacuations were saved if their strength was conserved appropriately. This was especially so if the bloodletting or induced vomiting or purging came at the onset. Many also

1 For the 1891 edition of the text based on this manuscript, see Pinkhof, *Abraham Kashlari*.

2 Dt. 2:36. Hayim Galipapa's lost chronicle of plague-related violence against Jewish communities invokes the same phrase. See Einbinder, *After the Black Death*, 80.

3 Paris, MS héb. 1191 has "on the fifth and seventh," which makes more sense.

4 They were continuous—i.e., the fevers.

5 Leiden, MS or. 4778—פרנשין; Paris, MS héb. 1191—פריני׳שין. Phrenitis, or frenesie, is a fever that affects the brain. Carpentieri and Mimura, "Arabic Commentaries on the Hippocratic Aphorisms"; Carpentieri, Fidora, and Lampurlanés, "Avicena y Gerardo de Cremona sobre la frenitis"; Jacquart, "Les avatars de la phrénitis."

6 Ferre, "Isaac Israeli's 'The Definition of Fever and Its Essence,'" section 34, translates as "mental disorder."

DOI: 10.17302/dohf20858 © Arc Humanities Press, 2026

expelled worms after purging and vomiting and they were saved from the anguish and fainting by either the purges or expulsion of the worms. In many of the afflicted, the signs of the fevers were confused: Sometimes symptoms of sanguine [fevers] were visible in redness of face, and sometimes those of phlegmatic [fevers][7] like lethargy and weakness,[8] sometimes those of choleric [fevers] like agitation, thirst, and dry mouth.[9] In many, the urine was clear, thin, and watery on the first day then thickened and reddened, and these [people] had severe headaches. In some, the urine turned white suddenly after days of being turbid and red. Because [the change] was sudden and acute, they had no hope in any physician or his art [of being saved] from death. The types of these fevers nearly eluded the physicians,[10] and their mixed signs led many to judge[11] them pestilential, so that they treated them for pestilential fevers and would feed them meat like poultry and wine **[fol. 115b]** at the onset and during the increase, and not bleed them, as they said this was how to treat pestilential fevers. But I saw that he who followed this regimen died. Still, there were those who were bled and evacuated and purged greatly, and these were saved, but a few died from loss of strength.

[Pinkhof, 50] Then wise and learned men requested I tell them my opinion for treating these fevers, and that I write this tractate. I fulfilled their wish and may any sage or such find it beneficial for these sicknesses if they occur. And may the benefit be for the present time and an example and model for those to come, as is the case for all the books that have been composed about this art, because it is concerned with individuals, for no man and his sickness is like another and therefore it is impossible that the individualized

---

7 Pinkhof has elided "in redness of face and sometimes those of phlegmatic."

8 אסטוטות, but compare Paris—אסטניסות, from the Greek, and in rabbinic Hebrew meaning "weakness."

9 Lit., dry tongue. Pinkhof has צמה ונגור הלשון, which should be emended.

10 Avicenna described pestilential fever rendering patients "hot to the touch" without any telltale change in pulse or urine until "suddenly they succumbed to a swift death." Aberth, *Doctoring the Black Death*, 114, citing the *Canon*, and see Avicenna, *Canon*, Book IV: 1.iv.2, which adds that the patient's sudden death confounds the physician. Aberth lists several physicians who remarked upon the baffling presentation of normal urine and pulse, including the Jewish physician Abraham b. Solomon Hen. According to Demaitre, the Montpellier university physician, Bernard de Gordon, also commented on the "deceptive" signs of pestilential fever, which preceded sudden death. Demaitre, *Medieval Medicine*, 64. Caslari associates the deceptive urine and pulse with fevers that are *not* pestilential: notice, however, that they are all describing the same clinical phenomenon.

11 Emending יפשטום to Paris's ישפטום.

formulations written in books will be well tempered for future individuals. Let them be **a measure and scale**[12] for the sage to add and detract according to his knowledge. I saw that if I did not make clearly known these fevers—what type they are—the truth of my opinion about their treatment would not be disseminated. Therefore, I have written briefly what is meant when we say pestilence and pestilential, and shall clarify their causes, signs, and treatment, after which I will make known my opinion about these fevers and their treatment.

CHAPTER: I thought intensely about these fevers and their signs, and I think that I have grasped matters that will serve the common good. I have written my opinion about what type they are and how they should be treated. Let the one who wishes study my tractate, whether he agrees or differs with my words: the signs lead directly to the truth.

SOME WILL CALL pestilence[13] or pestilential any sickness that spreads in a city, region, or districts and kills those who get it. They do not discriminate between those caused by an alteration in a quality of the air[14] generating a transmissible sickness or sicknesses—caused by over-exertion by the people of a household, city, or region, or the people of the city, region or regions consuming bad or unfamiliar foods, [**fol. 116a**] generating a transmissible sickness among the inhabitants—and [between] a transmissible sickness [caused] by corruption of the air and its poison-like putrefaction. They will call all these types pestilential. Indeed,[15] what is unique to the name pestilence or pestilential sickness that is called pestilence is that it is uniquely and by consensus a transmissible fever caused by air characterized by poison-like putrefaction and moist corruption that putrefies the vital spirit so that when continuously inhaled, the putrefaction suddenly reaches the heart, coming to mix with the heart's spirit quickly so that it heats up and generates continuous fevers that maintain putrefaction in the spirit. This putrefaction and corruption can be in a single household or a part of one, but it is possible for the putrefaction and corruption to be in a

12 Isa. 40:12.

13 Caslari uses the Hebrew word *dever* for pestilence. In its earliest, biblical usage, the term referred to an unspecified but collectively experienced disease event inflicted by God as chastisement. With the Black Death, it would become specifically associated with bubonic plague.

14 Condensing the Hebrew's "a change in the quality of the air from one of its qualities."

15 Following Lola Ferre, I read אמנם as equivalent to the Arabic "*imma*," an introductory emphatic.

great part of the land, a city or cities or districts and climates. But these sicknesses will only be generated in those predisposed [to them] who dwell in those places, and they will cause great and swift mortality. They will be very painful due to the putrefaction of the spirit in the heart, even though the putrefaction does not spread beyond the spirit. When this is so, the natural state of the urine shows little humoral alteration, nor does the pulse change much, nor is there pain in one of the members [**Pinkhof, 49**] because of the fever. Rather, their urine and pulse will be close to their natural state while the patient is already close to death due to corruption of the heart spirit, which is close to the soul that is the cause of life.[16] And if the putrefaction in the spirit is taken up into the humours or some of them by reason of the spirit's proximity and mixing with the humours,[17] fevers will be formed whose cause is putrefaction of the humours and spirit. Then the fevers will be humoral-pestilential, not pestilential, with signs of humoral fevers in the pulse, urine, and pain, and a change in the activity of the faculties distinct to the member for that humour and according to the humour that has putrefied. If it is in the brain, it will be a sanguine [fever]; the face will redden, the head will grow very heavy, with agitated lethargy,[18] confused imagination and hallucinations, if it is in the front of the brain. If it is in the middle chamber of the brain, confused wit and thought [will be present], and confused recall if it is in [**fol. 116b**] the back chamber of the brain. If it is sanguine in the stomach and liver, the appetitive and digestive faculty will be damaged, and the other faculties that serve the nutritive faculty. And thus[19] the faculties will be damaged according to the putrefaction of whichever humour in the member where the putrefied humour is [found].[20] The true physician-scholars have already written this in their tractates where any intelligent person can find it. That is not the intention of this essay, because my intention is only to clarify how those afflicted by what happened were[21] treated

---

16 Paris, MS héb. 1191 has "cause of the heat/fever."

17 Pinkhof's וערוכו should be emended to וערובו.

18 Hard to translate! The same term appears in Paris and is presumably technical. The patient is semiconscious or unconscious yet agitated?

19 Correcting Pinkhof's יוכן to וכן.

20 Emending to read the sentence without the final כאשר, which is missing in Paris and makes no sense in Leiden.

21 Compare Paris, MS héb. 1191's ינהגו, which yields "my intention is only to clarify how those afflicted by what happened should be treated with this regimen, and for any time that something similar occurs."

with this regimen, and for any time that something similar occurs; rather, we have presented this to clarify the fevers that occurred.

TRUE PESTILENTIAL FEVERS that are [caused by] a great, continuous putrefaction of the air that is poison-like [[in the air]]:[22] When it is inhaled, the heart spirit will be putrefied and grow hot. This heat is from bad, poisonous putrefaction that is not passed to the humours; it does not matter whether it is in one person or spreads among people. The CAUSES of these fevers: The general cause is putrefaction of the air with an alien heat and moisture that encompasses a certain area, whether inclusive or in part, in one or more climates, or in an individual place, a single city or household, or part of them, whatever the cause of the putrefaction. The causes of the fevers are terrestrial or celestial. The terrestrial will be [due to] proximity to putrefactions that corrupt the air, such as proximity to people with **severe leprosy, lepers, hectic fever and thirsting fever,**[23] who pass their corruption to the air and the operations. It can be [due to] proximity to many sicknesses, even those that are not transmissible. It can be proximity to plants and trees whose distinctive nature putrefies the air with pestilential putrefaction, as the empirics and testers agree.[24] This is apparent with BHYRH, like dates and nuts, especially when they fall and their leaves are rotten and corrupted. [It can be] in proximity to stinking water, rivers, aquifers,[25] and lakes that collect corruption, where linen is soaked[26] and the like—all the more so if there are corpses of poisonous animals and plants of bad, poisonous quality. [**fol. 117a**] Then transmission can take hold over a great or small distance and strengthen or weaken with respect to many or few, and

22 As noted above, double brackets indicate I have elided a dittography or redundancy, here the second "in the air." Single brackets enclose my additions.

23 Einbinder, *After the Black Death*, 81. Abraham partially cites Dt. 28:22 and adds lepers. The biblical Hebrew term *shiddafun* refers to agricultural blight, but in medieval medical Hebrew translates the Arabic *'istisqa*, or hectic fever. The term is used by Abraham's father, David, in his Galen translation; Bos et al., *Transmitting a Text through Three Languages*. *Gedemot*, from the Arabic *gudham*, refers to a leprous condition in which facial features and extremities disintegrate and fall off. See Avicenna's *Canon*, Book IV: 5.iii. *Tzara 'at*, also translated as leprosy, may signify an earlier stage or milder skin condition that was considered a distinct disease. *Kharkhur* is also a fever category, characterized by great thirst; *Canon*, Book V: 3.iii.

24 Lit., those who experiment and analogize—empirics and theorists?

25 חריצי-מים—See Rashi and Radak on Josh. 11:8, also B. Ketubot 79b; B. Shabbat 73b, and more.

26 משרת פשתן—Mishnah Berakhot 3:5 and its commentaries, which emphasize that the water stinks.

the strength or weakness, length or brevity, and duration of the corruption is what putrefies the air according to the susceptibility of places to receiving it.[27] [**Pinkhof, 48**] And the celestial CAUSE[28] is that the air will be putrefied at certain times, not through proximity to poisonous things that putrefy, [but] for celestial reasons, meaning when one of the planets harmful to us reaches places in its orbit that the Blessed One has ordained will have a harmful influence on our being and complexion, even if all God's deeds are good in themselves and of value to all existence. Since putrefaction of the air is a celestial cause, the fevers generated by this cause will be strong with sudden mortality due to the absence of prognosticating symptoms, confusing the physicians' knowledge of how to treat those who suffer from them [based on] science of the planets, their aspects and causes, until the matter, treatment, and prognosis is knowable only to astronomers, those who have investigated those celestial causes[29] that have occurred.

CHAPTER ON THE SIGNS OF THESE FEVERS: Their discernible signs were strong distress in the heart, [which is] not caused by pain because the increase of a humour is not sensible; blazing fever with ashen visage and a sudden loss of unificative faculty,[30] like someone who is exhausted by movement and feels weak until he appears to everyone in need of nourishment;[31] suppression of the natural heat to the spirit since the faculties are all carried in the spirit and when the spirits are suppressed, the faculties borne by them are weakened; and suppression of the distinctive vital motor faculty without fatigue or weariness in the members.

Most of what they experience is loss of appetite for food, confusion[32] from the suppression of the spirit in the brain that is sent to it from the heart,[33] [**fol. 117b**] also the spirit independently in the brain that is not

27 Rearranging the last two clauses so that "and [according to] the disposition for receiving it," which grammatically parallels the list of conditions beginning the sentence, comes at their end, and not following "the extension of the corruption..." where it sits in the text.

28 I follow Pinkhof's emendation of the text's הנהגה שמימית to סבה שמימית.

29 Emending Pinkhof's שפתבודדו to the manuscript's התבודדו still does not clarify the meaning. I defer to Paris's התבוננו, investigated or studied.

30 כח מנהיג, lit., directing or conducting faculty. According to Demaitre, *Medieval Medicine*, 20, the unificative faculty moves food to all parts of the body.

31 The manuscript reads עד שיראה הוא וכל המונו. I emend וכל to לכל.

32 Lit., "confused wits" (בלבול השכל).

33 The vital spirit.

brought from the heart,[34] as the guild of physicians explains; then they are afraid and dread death. Because there is no increase in humour, neither the urine nor its natural appearance deviates for the worse;[35] there may possibly be some change in agitation or sorrow or a cessation in eating. The pulse will not change as necessitated by an increase in humours deviating from equilibrium in quality or quantity, but it is possible that the urine and pulse will fluctuate as necessitated by the psychic operations when the spirit deviates from equilibrium.[36] Thus, their pulse and urine will be close to natural even as they are close to death, as [the putrefaction][37] reach[es] the heart and they draw near to death, so that the physician cannot predict their death from the signs in the urine and pulse ~~that would necessitate a change in the operations~~[38] and not from the few other natural symptoms in the body.

CHAPTER: ON THE PROGNOSTICATING SIGNS for these sicknesses:[39] Certainly, [for] those whose cause is air that is corrupted due to terrestrial causes [[that corrupt the air]] here are the signs of these causes: Certainly, for the pestilential fevers whose causes are celestial,[40] preceding these sicknesses the air appears to be [**Pinkhof, 47**] a foggy mixture from alien heat; heart constriction when breathing, as if [it were] heat from smoking wood,

34 The animal spirit.

35 Pinkhof emends the manuscript's דבר רע to דבר רק. I think the manuscript makes sense: there is no negative change in the patient's urine or appearance because there is no humoral excess.

36 The wording is difficult. Compare Paris's מחייב להפעיליות נפשיות to Leiden's המתחייב להפעיליות נפשיות. For different authorities on the relationship between the psychic operations and the pulse, see Nahyan Fancy, *Science and Religion in Mamluk Egypt: Ibn al-Nafīs, Pulmonary Transit and Bodily Resurrection* (London: Routledge, 2013), 105–8. The connection to the urine is unclear (to me). In Paris fol. 137b, the cause-and-effect relationship is reversed: the fluctuation in urine and pulse necessitate deviation of the spirit (and the psychic faculties?) from equilibrium.

37 Lit., "as they reach the heart," but comparison with Leiden fol. 137b clarifies that something is missing, namely that the prognosticating signs are not detected because the corruption or putrefaction reaches the heart so quickly.

38 Double dots over this phrase indicate deletion, bringing the wording close to that in Paris, fol. 137b.

39 Leiden and Paris share the same wording, but the signs associated with terrestrial causes are missing in Leiden. The passage moves directly to the signs for pestilence generated by celestial causes.

40 Pinkhof has elided "from corrupted air"—מאוירת בהפסד as superfluous; I agree.

a thick smoke;[41] and the leaves of plants detach[42] and fall before their time, the fruits putrefy quickly and animals flee from their nests, for the Creator Blessed be He imprinted in animals [the ability] to sense good air and flee from bad, corrupted air, especially several types of birds like the crow and its species, **the dove, swift and crane.**[43] When he sees these signs, the physician can prognosticate that the fevers will be pestilential. But experts in the laws of the planets know this from the laws of the planets, when the planets are in conjunction or eclipse, the laws of the seasons[44] as elucidated in that science. A physician cannot know this from being a master of the art of medicine, which only covers matters received from masters of the natural sciences and what is [**fol. 118a**] known in the science of medicine.[45] Their unique characteristics are that the urine and pulse remain natural or close to natural and there is great distress without an evident increase of humour in the stomach or other members, but the rest of the signs mentioned with the discernible signs of these fevers will surely always occur with humoral fevers.

CHAPTER: ON HUMORAL-PESTILENTIAL FEVERS. We've already said that the corruption from the putrefied spirit passes to the humours and is taken up by them. If one or more fevers are generated by them,[46] their signs will be those of another, non-pestilential fever like those of a particular humour, and that is because [the fever][47] is humoral but with some symptoms strengthened from its pestilential [aspects]. And when it is humoral-pestilential, the physician will be aided by their discernible and prognosticating signs; these will be more helpful for recognizing it. The urine and pulse and other signs and symptoms will be those of a humoral fever [event] [[from them]], as written in the books of the wise physicians. Because their humoral signs are shared with a few signs of pestilential fever, as we have said, which are great

---

41 The Hebrew is awkward. Compare Paris, fol. 137b, "as if it were the smoke of damp wood [that was] greatly damp."

42 Emending יותקו to ינתקו.

43 Jer. 8:7, "even the stork in the sky knows its seasons, **the dove, swift and crane** keep the time of their coming."

44 עתים. Seasons (or perhaps "cycles?")

45 See Aberth, *Doctoring the Black Death*, 63–67, on the physicians' attitudes toward astronomy/astrology.

46 Emending מהרה to Paris's מהנה.

47 Lit., "it."

pain[48] from the putrefaction of the spirit and loss of strength that occur in fevers for the elucidated reason [...].[49] But these are not a property of pestilential fevers, for these symptoms follow any putrefaction of spirit in the body for whatever reason,[50] but they are a symptom of an alien heat[51] whether the change is due to putrefaction of the spirit as in true pestilential fevers or [in] humoral-pestilential fevers in which the spirit is putrefied first and then the humour; or whether it is a putrefaction of the heart spirit due to its proximity to a putrefied humour that had putrefied first and then the putrefaction was taken up[52] by the spirit, as [happens] with non-pestilential fevers like *causon*,[53] phlegmatic and choleric humoral fevers; or due to emotional exertions like anger, grief, and others that change the complexion of the spirit. However, much of the distress in the fevers, and the rapid loss of strength for a[ny] reason not elucidated are characteristic of pestilential fever.

And not from the transmissibility of the bad fevers

[**Pinkhof, 46**] over a great area is there proof that they are pestilential, because transmission [**fol. 118b**] of diseases from a change in local diet to unaccustomed foods and the like is not among the causes for qualities of heat, cold, moisture or dryness [to be] generated in the air from non-putrefactive qualities. With a change in complexion there will be humoral fevers or altogether different sicknesses throughout the body or in a specific member.[54] When the cough or rheum[55] spread through a certain region,

---

48 מצוקה—pain, literally anguish or distress. Notice the difference in Paris, fol. 138a, which says these signs of pestilential fever are NOT what assists the physician in diagnosis, because the patient's pain and loss of strength are not necessarily acute and, in any case, these signs are not unique to pestilential fevers.

49 A phrase seems to be missing.

50 For whatever reason—lit., from whatever "side."

51 Eliding the following שוה רוח, which makes no sense.

52 Emending ונתחלק to Paris's ונתלקח.

53 דלקת, see Dt. 28:22; the term implies burning. *Canon*, Book IV: 1.ii.41: בקדחת השורפת ונקראת דלקת ובלשון יוני פאריטוש ובלשונם קבשון. In Book IV: 2.ii.35, *causon* is a subcategory of choleric fevers.

54 Convoluted, but clearer in Paris (fol. 138b) than Leiden. The fact that a disease is transmissible does not mean it is pestilential; diseases caused by irregular or unfamiliar diet are qualitative causes for a change of complexion that generates humoral fevers.

55 Following Lola Ferre's suggestion of "tos y rheume" for the otherwise enigmatic הרמד והשעול. Email message to author, November 28, 2024.

the change in humoral complexion damages their proportions,[56] disposing [people] to certain diseases, but pestilential sickness and pestilential air will not occur unless they have altered to a putrefied heat and moisture of a poisonous quality. But you should know that the humoral distress that is non-pestilential is from breathing the putrefied air, which is their distinctive and constant sign.

CHAPTER: THE REGIMEN for people during pestilence and the regimen for true and unadulterated pestilential fevers. [*Regimen for the fevers and the pestilential fevers*]. These are [the fevers] that occurred due to putrefaction of the air and its corruption, corruption and putrefaction of the spirit in the heart, not the humours. When you realize that the air is pestilential and the fevers pestilential from the signs we have indicated, attend to correcting the air and people's regimen with things that remove the putrefaction: That is, leave[57] the putrefied areas that are corrupting the air if the putrefied things are among the terrestrial causes we have indicated and correct the putrefied air with fumigations and foods from things that are cold, dry, and fragrant, and some drugs[58] that have putrefaction-removing properties, rendering the air quality impervious to putrefaction so that the terrestrial cause of putrefaction from the regions causing the corruption makes no impression[59] on the air. Even if the causes are celestial, these preparations will prevent the air from being impacted during a planetary flux. For an evil planetary flux will impact a person and place predisposed by nature to receive that flux, [**fol. 119a**] but will not impact those who are not, meaning those whose complexion opposes and diverges antithetically from to the flux. Were it not for this, all the people exposed to pestilential air would get pestilential illnesses from which they would die or recover during a time of pestilence. But that is not what happens. Rather, some sicken and some do not, and the reason is whether or not they are predisposed to receive that flux. Therefore, the air should be corrected with things that give the air a quality opposing the putrefaction, from the best things they can do to pestilential air accord-

56 ערכיהם—lit., values.

57 Reading תסיר as תסור, as per Leiden fol. 139a. The recommendation to flee an infected place was one of the most ubiquitous suggestions of medieval Christian and Jewish plague writing. For the complex Muslim response, see Stearns, *Infectious Ideas*.

58 Emending חמים to Paris's סמים.

59 Literally, it does not stamp or impress the air, but consequently also in the sense of "has/makes no impact."

ing to the regimens for health for treating these fevers and thus treating people with dietary regimens and scents whose fumigation makes an impression on the humours and spirits to make them opposed and antithetical to the putrefaction, until they prevent or limit their receiving an impression from the corrupting air. This is when they burn fragrant wood and multiply bonfires in pestilential places, especially fragrant woods and herbs[60] of myrtle and hyssop, pomegranate, juniper and citron and the other fragrant trees that counteract the putrefaction with the fragrance of their smoke and [**Pinkhof, 45**] destroy the putrefaction in the air. People should smell pomegranate leaves and the leaves of wild thyme[61] called *serpoll* dipped in vinegar. They should sprinkle places with crushed sandalwood, roses, and myrtle steeped in water and vinegar—10 parts each; frankincense—one part;[62] citron leaves, wild thyme leaves, and hyssop leaves—2 parts each; sprinkle them where the air is pestilential so they land on the stony and soft[63] areas in houses paved with stone floors—sprinkle them with what we have mentioned before, and especially when it is time to sleep when the faculties are dormant and will not oppose the bad qualities that are inhaled as they would when they are wakened and quick to actualize. This is the reason you prevent sleep in those bitten by poisonous [creatures], and those with poisonous apostemes, those who are choking,[64] or at the onset of the fever season. Their meals should have rooster and chicken, goat, calves, various types of small land and wild fowl, roasted, in soup or vinegar with pomegranate juice, unripe wine, lemon juice, and citron vinegar—no sheep, and those who eat pork should avoid it and be cautious with organ meat. [**fol. 119b**] They should also avoid fish except occasionally the red rock fish with scales, fried[65] with vinegar and hyssop, a little onion and Ceylonese cinnamon.[66] They should avoid waterfowl, and spices should be mostly

60 Emending עצי to עשבי.

61 Emending עשני נמאס ("smokes of wild thyme") to Paris's עלי נמאס ("leaves of wild thyme"); it may have once read עשבי נמאס, *nimās* herbs. *Nimās* is the Arabic for the Catalan *serpoll*, a type of wild thyme.

62 Correcting Pinkhof's לכונה to לבונה.

63 Paris fol. 139b has "stony areas and thresholds."

64 Literally, "choking," presumably referring to a disease that makes it hard to breathe or swallow (like diphtheria, whooping cough, pneumonia).

65 Or stewed?

66 דרציני—*dār tzini*, Ceylonese or Chinese cinnamon. According to Rosner, Maimonides and others used the term interchangeably for two different species, *cinnamomum zeylanicum* (found in Maimonides, Ibn Rushd, and others), and *cinnamomum cassia*.

Ceylonese cinnamon that is good and tolerable. He should avoid sweet fruits and especially dates, overripe squash and watermelon. He can eat sour, unripe fruits, which are tightening and astringent, like pomegranates, fragrant apples that are moderately scented, black plums, pears, and stewed fruits and apricots steeped in wine sauce; he should drink scented, mixed wine, smelling it, and he should avoid cheese and milk. He should begin his meal with a little onion in vinegar. Every morning, people[67] should drink fine white wine followed by a lemon electuary[68] weighing ½ scruple, which is ten grains of wheat, [and] *terra sigillata*. Alternatively, THIS RECIPE: take citron peel, fresh garden wormwood, hyssop, myrtle—an ounce each; Armenian bole, *terra sigillata*—a dram each; sugar—3 litras; rose water—½ litra; and make a drink; it will remove putrefaction and greatly strengthen the faculties and clarify[69] the spirits. They should concoct another drink after refining pure, pulverized, crystal—2 drams; garnet[70]—3 drams, [pome?]granate, clear and pulverized, wrapped in a white or red silk cloth, and they should always be stored in the jar for the potion. He should avoid scents that are greatly corrupting. THEY SHOULD EVACUATE the humoral excess from people; If there is a plethora in the blood, they should be bled;[71] and if there is an increase in one of the humours, they should be evacuated appropriately for fear of the putrefaction of the air being taken up in the superfluities in the humours and the spirits quickly [moving] to the natural moistures[72] whose

---

See Fred Rosner, *Moses Maimonides' Glossary of Drug Names* (Philadelphia: American Philosophical Society, 1974), 74, no. 95.

67 Note the sudden switch to the plural. Paris sustains the plural "they" throughout.

68 Electuary, for מרקחת, as per Michael McVaugh, Gerrit Bos, and Joseph Shatzmiller, *The Regimen Sanitatus of "Avenzoar": Stages in the Production of a Medieval Translation* (Leiden: Brill, 2019), sections 10, 11. 17, 24, 26.

69 יזהיר—lit., brighten.

70 אודם—garnet, or perhaps coral or ruby. A red stone. Coral acquired some traction as a plague prophylactic and as a prophylactic for children's diseases; see Nichola E. Harris, "The Protection of Innocents: Red Coral as a Lapidary Cure for the 'Children's Disease' and Conditions Related to Childbirth in Medieval and Early Modern England," in Lori Jones and Nükhet Varlık, eds., *Death and Disease in the Medieval and Early Modern World: Perspectives from Across the Mediterranean and Beyond* (Woodbridge: York Medieval/Boydell, 2022), 265–92. I am emending the meaningless חם to דר'.

71 Emending בכח הדם to בהם הדם, and יוזקו to יוקזו.

72 The entire passage is corrupt. Paris helps: see the parallel passage on fol. 140a. For יחקנה, Lola Ferre suggests emending to read יתקנה. I also emend מרה to read (as in Paris) מהרה, indicating that the corruption moves rapidly to the natural moistures. Alternatively, we could emend both copies to read מהנה, moving from the spirits to the natural moistures. Pinkhof has emended מרה ללחות to read מועילות, which still

purpose is to counter putrefaction. Smelling apple: sandalwood—the three [types],[73] plus cinnamon and balsam—one dram each; frankincense—½ oz.; camphor[74]; myrrh—100 grains; Sulphurwort[75]—3 drams; Ceylonese cinnamon—2 drams. They may be evacuated by this also. At night, use incense[76] when the house is shut, [**Pinkhof, 44**] and when fumigating, sprinkle the sprinkling water mentioned above.

CHAPTER FOR THOSE AFFLICTED BY UNADULTERATED PESTILENTIAL FEVER: If possible, remove them from that air, [**fol. 120a**] and if not, take the path mentioned in the preceding chapter, and turn to strengthening the heart with foods and therapeutic things, also with chickens roasted in sour things, lentil soup and white foods in lemon juice. They should limit their [consumption of] almonds and flours and drink white fragrant wine that is a little unripe,[77] pomegranate juice and citron vinegar steeped with *terra sigillata* and Armenian bole; he should eat soured fruit and particularly, moderately sweet pomegranates and apples, and plums ripened on the tree and unripe, sour mirobylans[78] and horseradish in vinegar. He should eat food [made with] rose juice and a compound of lemon juice, and smell

---

makes no sense, as the superfluity passing to the humours is a problem because it is putrefied, not because it resists putrefaction. The general meaning is clear: the danger of putrefaction passing from the air to the humours and from the humours to the moistures (in the heart or spirit) calls for evacuation of humoral excess.

73 See Paris. He is referring to three types of sandalwood.

74 There are many references to the use of camphor (Ar. *Kafūr*) in plague fumigants, sprays, and remedies. See Aberth, *Doctoring the Black Death*, ch. 3. *Kafūr* is amply documented in Arabic and Hebrew, e.g., in Oliver Kahl, trans. and ed., *Sābūr ibn Sahl* (Leiden: Brill, 2003); Claire Burridge, *Carolingian Medical Knowledge and Practice c. 775-900: New Approaches to Recipe Literature* (Leiden: Brill, 2024), 82n41 and elsewhere; Burridge says that camphor was imported to Carolingian Europe by the ninth century.

75 ארבאטור, in Paris עשב טור, *herbe tor*, *yerba tura*, or *hierba turis*. Lola Ferre, *Práctica de Johannes de Parma: Un tratado farmacológico en sus versiones hebreas y catalana* (Granada: Universidad de Granada, 2002), 71, 124, translates "hierba de incienso;" it may be related to frankincense. See also Gerrit Bos et al., eds. *Marwān ibn Janāh: On the Nomenclature of Medicinal Drugs (Kitāb al-Talkhīs)* (Leiden: Brill, 2020), 1:260–61, entry 56, under the Arabic "*andrāsiyun*," which the authors identify as sulphur wort or sulphurweed, also called hog's fennel.

76 Incense—מוגמר, relying on the translation of this term by McVaugh, Bos, and Shatzmiller, *The Regimen sanitatus of "Avenzoar,"* 144, 169.

77 Or, weak.

78 גדגדאניות—mirobylans. The word appears in the Hebrew translation of Ibn Wāfid's *Simple Drugs* with mirobylans as a synonym. There are multiple manuscript copies

"palace sandalwood," myrtle, and rose water steeped with camphor and saffron—a grain's weight each; white wheat—½ dram; ground cinnamon, balsam, fragrant myrtle—an ounce; rose water—a litra; boil it and put it in a silver vessel, or glass if silver is not possible, and dip white silk cloths in it and apply it to the face, nose and hands. Make compresses for the heart from white or red silk dipped in rose water as mentioned, a little *terra sigillata*, and apple juice and a little vinegar; limit [his] sleep. Evacuation of any sort with any purgative medicine is inappropriate, so as not to evacuate the spirit, which dissolves and dissipates in evacuation, especially for this fever, in the spirit that has been stunned by the turbulent pestilential air. An increase in humour does not require evacuation, because what is good and necessary for the body would be evacuated along with the spirit. Moreover, most purgatives contain something poisonous and contrary to a healthy complexion and to the heart's faculties. In no case let blood on the same side[79] for this fever, but if bloodletting is necessary, he should be bled from the opposite side after due consideration.[80] So, too, if an emetic is necessary, thus remove [?][81] act upon due and just consideration. Then let them drink this: AVOQDOLH, which is sorrel—a litra;[82] MSYNH;[83] sandalwood and rose water—a litra; fresh or dried violets stripped of their stems and pricks[84]—¼ litra; pomegranate juice steeped in wine—a ¼ litra each;

of the thirteenth-century Hebrew translation, הסמים הנפרדים; I used the fourteenth-century copy in Paris, BnF, MS héb. 1187 (IMHM F 15087).

79 Paris fol. 140a omits "on the same side."

80 Bloodletting should be from a vein on the opposite side of the affected area (the bubo, presumably), called revulsion, as opposed to derivation bleeding from the affected side. See Pedro Gil-Sotres, "Derivation and Revulsion: The Theory and Practice of Medieval Phlebotomy," in *Practical Medicine from Salerno to the Black Death*, ed. Luis García Ballester, Jon Arrizabalaga, and Roger French (Cambridge: Cambridge University Press, 1994), 110–55. Marie-Hélène Marganne, "Sur l'origine hippocratique des concepts de révulsion et de dérivation," *L'Antiquité classique* 49 (1980): 115–30; Voigts and McVaugh, "A Latin Technical Phlebotomy."

81 Probably a garbled distortion of Paris fol. 140b's רק מוצא הפרש, "just to remove the feces."

82 חמצאעת, and a few lines below, spelled חמצאניות. The term may refer to sorrel, which in Arabic is *humād*. Rosner, *Maimonides' Glossary of Drug Names*, no. 150, although the Castilian *labasa* and *acederilla* do not match Caslari's vernacular term. Found also below, where I have maintained the translation as sorrel despite its uncertainty.

83 Iris is Pinkhof's guess, reading משיכה. I read משינה, so I do not think so.

84 Violets as we know them do not have thorns or much stem. But when dried, flowers, stems and plant pieces become prickly, and stripping the flowers or leaves from stalks or stems, called garbling, can cause scratches and pricks as

myrtle juice—1 ½ oz.; [**fol. 120b**] sugar—3 litras. Make the drink and steep pure crystals, clear red stone,[85] pulverized—a dram apiece, wrapped in silk. Drink in water as desired. The sandalwood, violets, sorrel and silk should steep, crushed, for a day and night, then make the drink.

CHAPTER ON THE REGIMEN OF THOSE AFFLICTED WITH HUMORAL-PESTILENTIAL FEVERS: Know that there is no distinction between the regimen for those afflicted with these fevers and those afflicted with the other kinds of fainting-sanguine, [fainting]-choleric, or [fainting]-phlegmatic fevers, simple or compound.[86] The sanguine should be bled, and those with choleric and phlegmatic [fevers] should be purged; the humoral [fevers] should be treated with diets and medicines with care to the conditions of each. [**Pinkhof, 43**] The humoral-pestilential fevers should be treated with the regimen for humoral fevers. Attention to strengthening the heart must be greater than with non-pestilential [fevers], and he should attend to nourishing him more than he would for non-pestilential patients with foods suitable for a heart fever—even sometimes [with foods] that are not appropriate for fever but that taste better and are craved by the patient; treat so that the faculties are strengthened. He (the physician) should do this with oversight and intense study,[87] to feed [the patient] meat and well-blended fragrant wine, as the need for studying this is greater than the need for oversight concerning humour, spirit, and faculty. The physician should study the regimen for patients with humoral fevers and use it, then attend to overseeing the above-mentioned pestilential regimen with respect to correcting the air. I have left off mentioning this regimen in this essay because it was not my intention to clarify their regimen. Let him [the physician] draw from the treatises and commentaries that all the great men of this art have written.

---

if from thorns. My guess is that Caslari does not have a Hebrew word to describe "garbling." In Caslari's *Fresh Leaf*, violets are an ingredient in an emetic used to treat choleric fever. See, e.g., the version in Parma, PL, MS Cod. Parm. Heb. 1952, fol. 12a. In the *Antidotarium Nicolai*, they are cold and wet, drawing out bile and reducing inflammation, see Lola Ferre and Michael McVaugh, *The Tabula Antidotarii of Armengaud Blaise and its Hebrew Translation* (Philadelphia: American Philosophical Society, 2000), recipe nos. 6 and 9.

85 Again, a red stone (garnet? ruby? coral?); see note 70 above.

86 For varieties of fainting fever, see Avicenna, *Canon*, Book IV:1.ii.55–61.

87 השגחה ועיון. With oversight (clinical) and study (in books)? Perhaps, "oversight and scrutiny."

CHAPTER CONCERNING THE FEVERS THAT OCCURRED THIS YEAR: I wrote this essay especially to clarify the regimen for the fevers that occurred this year, their symptoms and accompanying signs, which were evident[88] even to ordinary people, let alone the sage physician. According to the signs, no sage would doubt that they were not true pestilential [fevers],[89] because they appeared with the signs and symptoms of humoral [fevers]. If there was any doubt, it was whether they were humoral-pestilential fevers or merely fainting-humoral, [**fol. 121a**] whose accompanying signs look similar, for pain and fainting increase with humoral-pestilential [fevers] and with humoral-fainting [fever] that is not pestilential. What resolves the doubt are the prognosticating signs drawn from the form of the air and whether or not it is pestilential, and whether pestilential causes preceded [them]. Certainly, the signs in the air were not evident in the spring or fall, not in fogginess or the rest; the flight of the birds from their nests and the crawling things from their holes; the fruits did not show more rot than usual according to their nature. Howsoever it was, it's the same whether they were fainting-humoral or humoral-pestilential [fevers], or even just humoral: they should be treated with bleeding or some other evacuation according to the increase in the putrefied humours. When I scrutinized[90] them in many people, they were compound, not simple, with an increase of blood and wateriness, great in ventosity and quantity, as if they were poisonous humours due to their great putrefaction and corruption [due to] their great quantity. Know that their qualities would rouse in the onset, overcoming nature. Thus, nature would be aroused against them at their onset to repel the humour and watery matter by means of sweat and fainting sweats. When it became thick at the extremity,[91] it could not purge with sweat or in the onset but would boil, rousing the matter to be shaken off by sweating, but the thickened matter would harden with boiling and not be purified. But if it happened that they [patients] were purified by purging, vomiting or strong bleeding, either during the remaining stages of the illness, independently or therapeutically, [**Pinkhof, 42**] they might be cured.

88 מפורסמים—lit., made known, disseminated.

89 Underlined in manuscript, but impossible to tell from the scans whether the underlining is original or was added by a later reader.

90 עיינתי. Caslari uses the same verb that I have translated as study or scrutinize.

91 "Thick at the extremity"of the blood vessel. The surfeit of inflamed humour cannot exit at the ends of the blood vessels because they are clogged, the build-up causes excess heat, and then it passes to the humoral sites outside the vessels.

That year, many presented with diarrhea, vomiting or great nosebleeds, but if their strength held up, many of them were cured. Some died from loss of strength due to the many evacuations and suddenness, even though it [evacuation] is appropriate according to the matter and its increase; this is like [what happens] to patients with many abscesses and excretions or dropsy[92] if the abscess or water is evacuated all at once, for the spirit bearing the faculties dissipates with the evacuated humour. The cause of these fevers may have been material, meaning bad dietary regimens, quantitative and qualitative, for there were high prices and [**fol. 121b**] shortages of the foods customarily eaten, **the five species of grain**,[93] so that most people were eating bread [made from] kernels and seeds that they were not used to, [from] fruit pips, chestnuts and acorns. It seems that the cause of the year's fevers was celestial; how the air and humours of non-pestilential quality generated entirely bad qualities in the humours.[94] It's true that Mars and the sun were in conjunction in the first degree from Aries and Mars is the planet that by God's will increases heat, burning, and boiling in the air and the humours, and the sun arouses heat and increases it. The sign and degree that were in conjunction there are the degree and sign of the aspect of Mars and its governances when it is at a maximum to rouse in the elements and their composites what they were created to rouse, namely heat, boiling, and burning.[95] It was when the sun set in Aries, which is the vernal equinox, that whatever planet would have governance that day would have governance for the entire year and especially in summer. Aries, which was in conjunction, guides sicknesses to the brain, and because there were heat and boiling, for this reason it (Aries) dominated the conjunction and with God's will necessitated the sicknesses that rise to the brain, like *birsām* and other sicknesses with boiling humours, [like] pox and measles.[96] God's will grants the planets and celestial bodies governance and influence on earth;

---

92 שקוי—dropsy. See Ferre, "Isaac Israeli's 'The Definition of Fever and its Essence,'" section 29; she says that David Caslari also used this term in his translation of Galen's *Peri Anomalou Dyskrasias*.

93 The rabbinic idiom for five species of produce refers to grain (Mishnah Challah 1:1; B. Talmud Berakhot 36b): wheat, barley, spelt, rye, oats.

94 The Hebrew is unclear; the translation is tentative.

95 The astrological alignment stirs up or rouses the elements and what is created or compounded from them to cause heat, boiling, and burning.

96 בגדרי וחצבה—Arabic for smallpox and measles. Avicenna describes them as fevers caused by the boiling of choleric humour, as Caslari indicates; the boiling causes putrefaction. See the *Canon*, Book IV: 1.iv.7–8.

then qualities in the lower world are created in the elements and their composites that generated these sicknesses and fevers on earth in places and among people predisposed to receive them, to whomever the Most Blessed God brought them. Even though the study of celestial causes and properties does not belong to the physician's domain except to the degree he is an astrologer or a metaphysician and Torah scholar, I saw fit to mention this cause because some would-be sages boasted and said that the sicknesses were pestilential because the conjunction required it. But even though they were transmissible sicknesses, and the conjunction may have contributed to their emergence, not every transmissible sickness or what is determined by a conjunction or planetary influence is pestilential. Nor do the laws of the planets require that this conjunction be followed by the generation of true pestilential qualities, which we have defined, [**fol. 122a**] unless God wills the boiling and burning of the humours and the rise of sicknesses to the higher members.

[**Pinkhof, 41**] **THE REGIMEN FOR THE FEVERS THAT OCCURRED**: For those that were all of one type and similar symptoms [affecting] different faculties, it is most appropriate to relieve their stomach at the onset to eliminate the feces, whether by means of emetics [or] by eating laxative, releasing foods from releasing vegetables with some purgative [value] like beets, *mercurialis annua*,[97] QVSYS and some corriola,[98] scalded in water with a little oil of crushed violets in vinegar, juice of pomegranates and unripe grapes. Let him drink from their broth and eat the vegetables. If[99] they relieve [him], good. If not, let him be relieved with this: Let him be given an emetic on the second evening, and even better on the first, second, and third. Let him be bled from the median or cephalic vein in the right or left arm as the physician gauges best, and bleed him in moderate quantity, according to the person and his custom, strength, and complexion. If he is a youth, scratch behind the ears, and if his head aches greatly from all the purging and bloodletting, then letting blood from the north would be good. On the fourth day,

---

97 In the *Fresh Leaf*, it appears in an emetic for sanguine fever. I think it is *mercurialis annua*; see Aberth, *Doctoring the Black Death*, ch. 3, and en.wikipedia.org/wiki/Mercurialis_annua. Although varieties of the plant are toxic, it found medicinal use as a laxative and, according to Wikipedia, as a wound salve among Native Americans.

98 Or corregiola, corregüela in modern Spanish. There are two varieties, *libleb kabīr* and *libleb sagīr*, large and small convolvulus (which are actually different plants). A diuretic and expectorant, *libleb* appears in Caslari's *Fresh Leaf* for treating sanguine fever. Rosner, *Maimonides' Glossary of Drug Names*, 144.

99 Pinkhof dropped the passage between "scalded" and "if."

let him be purged with a purgative containing violets, prunes, Indian dates, *mana nār*, pine nuts[100] and rhubarb, all or a few of them as the physician gauges fitting. If he sees fit to apply polipode,[101] let him do so, for this purgative treats all the humours, which are all mixed together in these sicknesses, and it is light, not cutting all the faculties, for it contains nothing purging of bad or poisonous quality. Morning and evening, wash their thighs and legs briskly with a concoction of willow leaves, grape vine, and chamomile, and if nonetheless their head still aches and there are signs that the sickness is rising to the head, and five or six days have passed with adherence to the regimen, perhaps the faculties have weakened too much for a general bloodletting. [Then] apply leeches to the forehead and nose, and bleed from the veins under the tongue. Or bleed his nose, shave the head and wash it with a concoction of NPYM and cooling things with a little repulsion; let them [the ingredients] be balanced according to the physician's judgment. Roses—3 oz., curcumin—1 1/2 oz.; chamomile and meliote—an ounce apiece; this is suitable [**fol. 122b**] at the beginning of the increase of the sickness, repelling the rising vapours, dissolving the fumigating vapours that have arisen, cooking, numbing[102] and quieting the pain. This is done after evacuating them[103] if the pain is strong, with horseradish juice and rose water, equal amounts of each; vinegar—one in twenty. If [he is] greatly agitated even so, apply this ointment to their forehead after the washing: rose,[104] PVPVLYON—an ounce each; oil YBRVKh—½ oz.; chamomile oil—1 ½ oz.; wax—1 oz.; with saffron—½ dram; white wax—an oz.; make an ointment. Feed him with beverages cooked with melon seed milk, and limit milk of almonds, especially old ones, which are hot and add [excess] to the mid-brain, causing it pain. Alternatively, feed him with lentil or chickpea soup ~~with a little lentil soup or chickpea soup~~[105]with a little parsley[106] and vinegar, cooked pumpkin, and the vegetables mentioned above; do not put any borage in the foods. Plums,

100 שנבר

101 Or bisbeige, and "polipodio" in Ferre, *Práctica de Johannes de Parma*, 11, 13/45, and 37/25.

102 מישן—putting to sleep.

103 Reading אחרי חקוקן as אחרי חקונן

104 A variety of rose? ורדיית rather than the usual ורד.

105 The repeated phase is dotted for elision.

106 Emending Pinkhof's פוטר to פיטר throughout. See Ferre and McVaugh, *The Tabula Antidotarii*, no. 36; also in Ferre, *Práctica de Johannes de Parma*. Pinkhof thought the word referred to a mushroom (as in פטריות) but it must be parsley (as in petrosilla).

fragrant apples, horseradish, citron, and portolaca[107] YVPLV in them. The air should always be corrected with a bit of cooked myrtle and grapes, grape leaves, sweet cane,[108] and a little citron leaf. Always close the windows on the east and south; their arms and [**Pinkhof, 40**] hands should be bathed in warm water, which greatly helps pain in the heart on whichever side. After being bathed in hot [water], the[ir] hands should be dried and put in cold water. Let hot water be mixed with young mulberries, a little vinegar and rose water. On their hearts, always put grape leaves steeped **IN THIS**: Rose water—½ litra; white wine—an oz.; vinegar—an oz.; saffron—½ a simple mithqal;[109] camphor—a wheat seed's weight; sandalwood—all a ½ dr.; a decoction of myrtle—2 oz. should be mixed in. Know that he should greatly avoid meat and wine, unless it is necessary for fear of a loss of strength, which [strength] may be reinforced by eating what is familiar and craved more than [it is] by medically indicated foods that strengthen but are unfamiliar and that he does not crave. A DRINK for morning and evening. It is a therapeutic food that releases; it strengthens the heart, [**fol. 123a**] kills and expels the worms that were common with the sicknesses of this year, and corrects the humours and prepares them for purging, urinating and sweating: Sorrel, fiddle dock haAGUDAH,[110] maidenhair fern,[111] garlic root, parsley, asparagus root—¼ litra apiece; skin of mulberry root—½ litra; wormwood bark, citron peel, sumac—½ oz. each; *fumus terre*[112]—an oz.; endive juice,

---

107 Portolaca–myrobylan. See Ferre, "Isaac Israeli's 'The Definition of Fever and its Essence,'" 26, 33; Ibn Wāfid's compendium of simple drugs identifies חלילג as myrobylan and says there are four types; again, I used the copy of הסמים הנפרדים in BnF, MS héb. 1187, fol. 14a.

108 Sweet cane—a kind of lemongrass; see קנה טוב in McVaugh, Bos, and Shatzmiller, *The Regimen sanitatus of "Avenzoar,"* 146 Hebrew and 174 English. A variety of cinnamon is also possible.

109 Eight mithqāls (an Arabic measure)—1 oz.

110 לפאס האגודה. I tentatively identify LPAS with the herb known in Spanish as lampaza, acedera, lapazuela etc., Catalan arengada, collerosa etc. See Ferre, *Práctica de Johannes de Parma*, 67, with the Hebrew spelling לאפסה. The scientific name is *Rumex pulcher*, in the Polygonaceae family. Medicinal uses include treatment for diarrhea, constipation, stomach cramps, and tumors. Colloquially in English the plant is called fiddle dock or bitter dock, whose leaves contain high levels of oxylic acid that gives them a bitter lemon taste; see pfafol.org/user/plant.aspx?LatinName=Rumex+pulcher. The Hebrew AGUDAH could refer to a bunch or bundle?

111 *Capillus veneris.*

112 Fumus terre, fumaria, fumitory juice. See Ferre, *Práctica de Johannes de Parma*, 9, 27; Ferre and McVaugh, *The Tabula Antidotarii*, 10, 56.

bindweed juice—a litra each; camphor juice, *mercurialis annua* juice—½ litra each; violet—1/4 litra; juice of roses preserved in sugar, lemon juice, *diamente*[113]—2 oz. each; vinegar—½ oz; sour citron juice—an oz. per litra; sugar—1 litra; it should be fully decocted. If the sick person has been relieved, remove the juice of bindweed, camphor and *mercurialis*: Substitute rose water for the rose extract and steep ½ oz. of red sandalwood in the drink; SYS—3 dr. Adults should drink [it] in the morning with 4 ½ oz. hot water cooked with chickpeas [and] mastic. For children, two spoonfuls for ten days[114] in which a little mastic or sumac have been cooked.

The TYREAN OINTMENT:[115] His stomach should be anointed with this if the Tyrean [ointments] are not prepared: wormwood oil, oil of bitter almonds, ½ oz. cocted sumac and ½ oz. citron peel, a dram of SYNTONYQA, vinegared pomegranate juice—3 oz. each. Cool together until it is like an oil. White wax—an oz., aloe[116]—½ oz., and make an ointment.

ROSE OINTMENT: rose water or juice—½ litra; papaver juice—a ¼ litra each;[117] if juice cannot be found, substitute cocted papaver seed in 2 litras water until it is reduced to a half-litra. Seed oil or pumpkin seed oil—a litra; chamomile oil—¼ litra. Let the oil be cooked with the above-mentioned until the oil alone remains on the embers. Then crush white wax—3 oz., and remove from the fire until it crumbles, add saffron powder, opium powder—a simple mithqal.

A TYREAN OINTMENT: We use [this] for poisonous [things] [**fol. 123b**] and for snakes,[118] for worms in the stomach and other members. Take juice of centaura[119]—large and small; wormwood juice; apricot leaf, portolaca juice, QRYSPYVNL juice, vinegar, citron nectar, lemon juice—a litra each; half of it should be mixed, dried, and pulverized, mixed with oil to make a paste: lupin[120] flour—a litra; cinnamon, frankincense, myrrh—an oz. each; aloe,

---

113 A mint compound. Personal correspondence, Michael McVaugh, October 2024.

114 Or, as Pinkhof has emended, "two spoonfuls in ten of water."

115 Aberth, *Doctoring the Black Death*, 180, refers to a "Tyrean saffron" that was both toxin and antidote, and used as a plague prophylactic.

116 צבר. See Ferre and McVaugh, *The Tabula Antidotarii*, no. 57.

117 An ingredient must be missing, as we have only the papaver here. Papaver is the plant from which opium, morphine, and heroin are derived.

118 Following the brilliant suggestion of my anonymous reader to emend ליחשים to לנחשים. Thank you, anonymous reader!

119 סנטוריאה—*centaura*, a purging drug. See Ferre, *Práctica de Johannes de Parma*, 37. Often used with polipode.

120 לופינש—lupin, here as flour and perhaps from the legume seeds, which are

balm—½ oz. each; ox gall[121]—an oz.; peel of mulberry root [**Pinkhof, 39**] and pomegranate, sumac, cleaned citron seeds; peel of root of PLGYRV, SYNTONYQA seed of ALYSSNDRA;[122] carob seed; rue—½ oz. each; peel of dried citron, fine[ly diced]—3 oz.; *terra sigillata*; burnt stag horn—an oz.: Mix well with powder the juices [of] violets with aloe, balm, and myrrh powder suitable for pulverizing; take almond oil, apricot oil—4 litras each; rose extract (oil), mastic oil, nard—3 oz. each; wax—½ litra. Let it solidify and mix well with the powdered ointment mentioned above.

FINISHED AND COMPLETED, PRAISE TO THE ETERNAL GOD.

edible. The flowering stalk is colloquially known as bluebonnet.

121 מררת פר—ox gall, cow's bile or gall. It is used in papermaking (to marble paper) and lithography; in traditional Chinese medicine it was used to expel worms and treat jaundice. Caslari refers to expelling worms as an effect of the Tyrean ointment in the immediately preceding recipe, so this may its purpose here, too.

122 *Alissandre*: I do not know what this is, but this is clearly the transcription.

TRANSLATION OF PARIS, BIBLIOTHÈQUE NATIONALE DE FRANCE, MS héb. 1191, fols. 134b–141a

ABRAHAM B. DAVID CASLARI, *TRACTATE ON PESTILENTIAL FEVERS AND FEVER TYPES*

NLI, IMHM F 14747

[**fol. 134b**] Said the son of the enlightened David, his son Abraham, father of the sage Yehacel Caslari: I was moved to compose this tractate by what happened in the summer and late spring; fevers encompassed all the region of Provence, all Catalonia and Aragon—**not a city or town was spared** by the fevers,[1] and especially the sanguine youths of good regimen, and the fevers killed them. Not eleven days would pass, and many died on the fifth and seventh. They were continuous fevers without intermittence, with much fainting and anguish. Some would commence with shivering and strong fever; the sick person sweated greatly on the first day, after which the fever strengthened and remained continuous. They sweated on the third and fifth [days] and were continuous even on the seventh; they also sweated with great anguish—many of them died in anguish. For many, the matter rose to the head, with phrenitis[2] and mental confusion. Many who grew weak then experienced weakness in the limbs and died. Many experienced nosebleeds, or for women a release of vaginal blood, or vomiting or strong diarrhea. [If they were] bled and purged with medicines, many who had one of these evacuations were saved, all the more if their strength was conserved appropriately. This was especially so if the evacuation of blood or vomit was at the onset, or the purge. Many also expelled worms after purging, and the expulsion of worms was due to anguish and fainting. In many of the afflicted, the signs of the fevers were confused: Sometimes symptoms of sanguine [fevers] were visible in redness of face, and sometimes those of phlegmatic [fevers]

1 Dt. 2:36. Strikingly, the Paris version omits Castile and Navarre, both included in the plague's trajectory recorded in the Leiden text. The Black Death reached Besalú in the spring of 1348 and Castile late in 1348 or early in 1349, which could place the original source of the Paris text prior to Caslari's knowledge of the plague's arrival in Castile. Einbinder, *After the Black Death*, 88.

2 Leiden, MS or. 4778—פרנישין. Phrenitis, or frenesie, a fever category characterized by hallucinations and mental confusion. Carpentieri and Mimura, "Arabic Commentaries on the Hippocratic Aphorisms;" Carpentieri, Fidora, and Lampurlanés, "Avicena y Gerardo de Cremona sobre la frenitis;" Jacquart, "Les avatars de la phrénitis."

DOI: 10.17302/dohf20859

like lethargy and weakness, sometimes the sign of [**fol. 135a**] choler in agitation, thirst, and dry mouth. The urine of many of the afflicted was clear, thin, and watery on the first and second day, then it thickened, reddened and grew turbid, and they had severe headaches. Because [the changes] were sudden and acute, they had no hope in any physician or his art [of being saved] from death. The types of these fevers nearly eluded the physicians. Many judged them pestilential and treated them according to the regimen for pestilential fevers, so that many physicians fed them light meat, especially poultry, and permitted them wine at the onset, increase, and duration; they would not evacuate them, as they would say this was how to treat pestilential fevers. But I saw that most of those who followed this regimen died. Yet there were those whom they would bleed and purge and most of them were saved, although a few died from loss of strength.

Then wise and learned men requested that I tell them my opinion of these fevers and how to treat them. I saw that if I did not make clearly known the definition of these fevers and what type they were, the truth of my opinion about their treatment would not be disseminated. Therefore, I have written briefly what is meant when we say pestilence or pestilential, and shall clarify their causes, signs, and treatment. Afterwards, I shall give my opinion about the fevers that occurred and their treatment, with the help of God.

CHAPTER: Abraham said: I thought deeply about these fevers and their signs, until I think that I have grasped their matter, and I am writing my reasoning about what type they are and how they should be treated for the common good. He who wishes to know my opinion, according to my reasoning, let him agree or disagree with me; the signs lead to the truth. For introduction, I will clarify and define the term pestilence.[3] There are those who call pestilence any illness that kills suddenly and [**fol. 135b**] spreads in a city, region, or districts. There is a difference between corruption of the air due to putrefaction and that which is due to bad diet, fatigue or exertions that deviate from what had been [people's] customary regimen, then fever emerged among them for this reason. But what is unique to the term pestilential fever is that they are fevers whose cause is air characterized by putre-

3 Caslari uses the Hebrew *dever* for pestilence. The biblical term referred to an unspecified but collectively experienced disease event inflicted by God as chastisement. With the Black Death, it would become specifically associated with bubonic plague.

faction, due to the ease with which it is activated[4] in proximity to rotting things and corpses, also plants and trees that have the property of putrefying the air with a pestilential putrefaction, like the date, nut, and cabbage, all the more when their leaves fall and rot. Also, proximity to fetid waters, stagnant water, and soaking linen will impress putrefaction on the air that will putrefy the bodies that are predisposed to receive that activation and corruption of heat, moisture, and putrefaction. Due to constant inhalation, the vital spirit mixes with the spirit in the heart, becomes heated and generates continuous fever because of the continuing putrefaction in the spirit. This putrefaction and corruption can be in a single household or part of one so that sicknesses only emerge among those who dwell in that house. [Or] the putrefaction and corruption can be in a large part of the land, a city or cities, and then the pestilence will be found among the residents of that place who are predisposed to it. Those fevers will be very painful, because the heart spirit is putrefied even though the putrefaction has not spread to the humours but is only in the spirits. When this is so, the urine will hardly change its natural colour, because there is no change in the humour. The pulse will also not be greatly changed, nor will there be pain in one of the members. Among these it happens that the urine and pulse will be close to natural [**fol. 136a**] but the sick person is close to death due to the corruption of the spirit in the heart, which is a proximate instrument to the soul which is the cause of the heat.[5] If perhaps the putrefaction is taken up from the spirit to the humours or to part of them due to the spirit's proximity and mixing with the humours, the cause of the fevers will be their putrefaction and corruption. Then the fevers will be humoral [with regard to] urine and pulse; the pains and change in the activity of the faculties distinct to the member where the humour has taken up the putrefaction, and the members containing that humour, will be symptomatic of the humour that has been putrefied. FOR EXAMPLE, if it is in the brain, it will be sanguine, the eyes will redden, the face will swell and redden, there will be great pain in the head, and agitated lethargy,[6] with confusion of the imagination and hallucination if in the front of the head and sleepiness or mental confusion.[7] If the humour is sanguine in the stomach and liver, the appetitive and digestive faculty will

---

4 מצד קלות התפעלותו

5 Leiden has "cause of life" (סבת החי as opposed to סבת החום).

6 Leiden uses the same expression, which must be technical.

7 Bos et al., *Transmitting a Text Through Three Languages*, translate the term as "mental disorder," or "melancholy, madness."

be damaged, and the other faculties that pass through[8] the nutritive faculty. Thus, the faculties will be damaged according to the putrefaction of each humour in whatever member the humour has been putrefied.

THE TRUE scholars[9] have already written about this in their essays, where any sage can find it. Our clarification in this treatise is not intended [to treat this], because my intention is only to clarify how to treat those afflicted with fevers at the time of the episode that befell them this year; it may also be beneficial for every time and place that something similar happens according to the above-mentioned signs.

CHAPTER: A TRUE PESTILENTIAL FEVER is that which is [caused by] a bad, continuous putrefaction of the air that is poison-like [[in the air]]:[10] When it is inhaled, the heart spirit will be putrefied and grow hot with an alien heat from a bad putrefaction that is not passed to the humours; it does not matter whether it is in one person or spreads among people.

The causes of these fevers [136b]

The general cause is putrefaction of the air with an alien heat and moisture that encompasses a certain area, whether it includes a large portion of a climate or climates, or is in an individual place like a single city or household, or part of them, whatever the cause of the putrefaction. *The causes of the fevers are both terrestrial and celestial.* The TERRESTRIAL would be proximity to people with **severe leprosy, lepers, hectic fever and thirsting fever,**[11] whose corruption mixes with the air with its quick action.[12] It can also be proximity to corpses and rotting bodies, also proximity to starving people whose breath is corrupted. It can also be proximity to plants and

8 Pass through (עוברים); perhaps an error for "serve" (עובדים): the faculties that serve the nutritive.

9 Lit., חכמי המחקר, sages of research or investigation.

10 Eliding the reiterated "in the air." As noted above, double brackets indicate my elisions. Single brackets indicate my additions.

11 Einbinder, *After the Black Death*, 81. Abraham echoes Dt. 28:22, adding lepers. The biblical term *shiddafun* refers to agricultural blight but in medieval medical Hebrew, it translates the Arabic *'istisqa*, or hectic fever. The term is used by Abraham's father, David, in his Galen translation; Bos et al., *Transmitting a Text through Three Languages*. *Gedemot*, from the Arabic *gudham*, refers to a leprous condition in which the facial features and extremities disintegrate and fall off. See also Avicenna, *Canon*, Book IV: 5.iii. *Tzara'at*, also translated as leprosy, may signify an earlier stage or milder skin condition that was considered a distinct disease. *Kharkhur* is a fever characterized by great thirst; *Canon*, Book V:3.iii.

12 Leiden has "who pass their corruption to the air and its operations," fol. 116b.

trees whose distinctive nature putrefies the air with pestilential putrefaction, as the empirics and testers[13] agree. This is evident with proximity to dates, nuts, and cabbage when their leaves fall and are corrupted.[14] It can also be proximity to stinking waters, rivers, aquifers,[15] and lakes that collect corruption, where linen is soaked[16] and the like, all the more so if there are corpses of poisonous animals and plants of bad, poisonous quality. Then transmission can occur over a great or small distance and [strengthen][17] or weaken with respect to many or few, and the strength or weakness, length or brevity, and duration of that putrefied corruption [is what] putrefies the air according to the susceptibility of places to receiving it.

THE CELESTIAL [cause] is when at times the air is putrefied, without proximity to earthly things that are putrefying.

The celestial cause: This means when one of the planets that is harmful to us reaches a place in [its] orbit that the Blessed One has ordained to have a harmful influence on human complexion and poisons it, or to a conjunction of harmful planets causing influences that are toxic to [**fol. 137a**] the air with respect to our constitution and complexion, even though it is surely true that all God's actions are good in themselves and with respect to all existence.[18] Since the cause of the air's putrefaction is celestial, the fevers it consequently generates will be strong and death will be sudden, lacking pain among the symptoms, contradicting the prognostication of the physicians and confusing them[19] about how to treat the sufferers according to knowledge of the planets and the place of their aspects and conjunctions, until their substance, treatment, and prognosis of their outcome are not understood except to masters of astronomy, those who have studied the verification of the celestial cause that has occurred.

---

13 Who exactly is meant by "testers" I do not know. Empirics? Pharmacists? Herbal experts?

14 Presumably, rotten.

15 חריצי-מים See the medieval exegetes Rashi and Radak on Josh. 11:8; B. Ketubot 79b; B. Shabbat 73b and more.

16 משרת פשתן—see Mishnah Ber. 3:5 and commentaries, which emphasize that the water stinks.

17 "Strengthen" is found in Leiden, fol. 117a, and was apparently dropped here.

18 Lit., "reality" (מציאות).

19 The same term was used above to describe "mental confusion."

The accompanying SIGNS: strong distress in the heart, not due to pain, because there is no increase in humour there, [but] he will feel burning heat, have an ashen visage and a sudden loss in the unificative faculty, so that his movement is listless and he feels weak until it seems to all[20] that he is in need of strengthening; and suppression of the natural heat to the spirit since the faculties are all carried in the spirit and when the spirits are suppressed[21]the faculties borne by them are weakened, especially the vital motor faculty that is in the heart. There will be fatigue and weariness in the members, and most will experience loss of appetite for food, confusion from the suppression of the spirit that is sent to the brain from the heart, or from the spirit itself without it being brought from the heart, as the guild of physicians explains. They will experience corruption and dread of death. Neither the urine nor its natural appearance will change for the worse because there is no increase in humour; some change may occur if he is agitated [**fol. 137b**], sad or stops eating. The pulse will also not change as necessitated by an increase of humours deviating from equilibrium in quality or quantity. It is possible that the urine and pulse cause fluctuation[22] in the psychic operations and deviation of the spirit from equilibrium. Thus, the pulses and urines of these people will be close to normal even though they are close to death, as if they were bitten or stung by something poisonous, because the change in their humours will not be manifested and their signs will not be recognized because of the suddenness with which [the poison-like corruption] reaches the heart, nor their imminent death. Thus, the physician is unable to predict their death from the signs in the urine and pulse, nor from other natural symptoms in the body.

CHAPTER: On the prognosticating signs for these sicknesses

Certainly, [for] those whose cause is air that is corrupted due to terrestrial causes [[that corrupt the air]] here are the signs of these causes:[23] Certainly,

---

20 Emending וכל המזג' to Leiden's וכל המונו.

21 Emending תרעבנה to Leiden's תדעכנה.

22 The wording is difficult. Compare Paris's מחייב להפעיליות נפשיות to Leiden's המתחייב להפעיליות נפשיות, fol. 117a. For different authorities on the relationship between the psychic operations and the pulse, see Fancy, *Science and Religion in Mamluk Egypt*, 105–8. The connection to the urine is unclear (to me). Leiden's account seems to say that the psychic operations produce the fluctuation in the urine and spirit, while Paris says the reverse.

23 Leiden and Paris share the same convoluted wording. Both copies also fail to list the signs for pestilential fevers with terrestrial causes but move directly to the signs associated with celestial causes.

the pestilential fevers that are formed due to celestial causes that cause a corrupt quality in the air [are such that] preceding the sicknesses, the air will appear mixed with fog and alien heat that is painful[24] when inhaled [is] like smoke from very damp wood. Also, the leaves of the plants will detach and fall off when it is not time for them to do so. The fruits will putrefy quickly, and animals will flee from their resting places and birds from their nests,[25] for the Creator has impressed in birds and animals a sense of the airs and how to choose good air and to flee from bad, putrefying, and corrupting airs, especially a few kinds of birds like the types of crow, swift, and crane.[26] When he sees all or a few of these signs, the physician can prognosticate that the fevers will be pestilential. Certainly, experts in the laws of the planets **[fol. 138a]** will know this from the laws of the planets, their conjunctions, eclipses and the laws of the seasons as elucidated in that science. However, a physician cannot know this from being a master in the art of medicine, because the science of medicine does not go beyond what is accepted by experts in natural science and known to the science of medicine.[27]

CHAPTER: When a fever is accompanied by diarrhea that is dissolved and soft, that fever is pestilential, because that is a symptom that is not absent from pestilential fevers.[28]

CHAPTER: *On the humoral-pestilential fevers*

We've already said that when the putrefaction of the spirit is continuous, its corruption will pass to the humours and be taken up by them. If this creates one or two or more fevers, their signs will be like the signs of another, non-pestilential, fever that is constituted like those of a particular humour, and that is because [the fever] is humoral but with some symptoms strengthened from its pestilential [aspects]. When it is humoral-pestilential, the physician will be aided by their discernible and prognosticating signs [which] will help in recognizing it. The signs from the urine and pulse and other symptoms will be like those of a humoral fever event, as has been written in

24 Or constricting.

25 See Avicenna, *Canon*, Book IV: 1.iv.3.

26 Notice that the author or copyist has altered the "dove, swift and crane" found in Leiden fol. 117b and citing Jer. 8.7. At the same time, he has inserted an elegant pun by saying that the birds know how to "choose" (בחר) good air and flee (ברח) from bad.

27 Compare Leiden fol. 117b.

28 Missing in Leiden and not obviously organic to the discussion here. It could have been added by a later copyist who had already experienced subsequent plague outbreaks.

the books of the wise physicians. It is not necessary[29] for the humoral signs to be accompanied by a little pestilential quality, which as we have said are great distress from the putrefaction of the spirit, a rapid loss of strength and such, because the distress is not intense, and the loss of strength that occurs in fevers for the elucidated reason does not [just] characterize pestilential fever, for symptoms like these follow any putrefaction of spirit in the body from whatever reason. Rather, they are a symptom of an alien heat that [**fol. 138b**] reaches the heart, whether [due to] the complexion of his strength or due to putrefaction of the spirit alone, as in true pestilential fevers; or [to] a fever in which the spirit is putrefied first and then the humour; or whether the cause is a putrefaction of the heart spirit[30] due to its proximity to a putrefied humour that had putrefied first and then the putrefaction was taken up[31] by the spirit; as in the non-pestilential phlegmatic and choleric humoral fevers; or from psychic exertion as from anger, grief, and sadness, and other exertions that alter the spirit. Certainly, great distress in the fevers and rapid loss of strength for a[ny] reason not elucidated are characteristic of pestilential fever. That the fevers spread over a great area is not proof that they are pestilential, for the transmissibility of diseases is not a property of pestilence but occurs for all sicknesses [caused by] diet, change of location, and people eating foods they are not accustomed to and the like, from reasons [to do with] qualities that are not pestilential.[32] The change in their complexion causes humoral fevers or other sicknesses throughout the body or in a specific member. One year cough and rheum[33] will spread through a certain region because of an alteration in humoral complexion and damage to their[34] proportions, so they will be disposed to receive certain sicknesses. [We] do not call sicknesses or air[35] pestilential unless they

29 Compare Leiden fol. 118a, which says that the fevers do carry some pestilential signs, but signs that accompany all fevers characterized by putrefaction of spirit. The visual similarity of ולא (Paris) and ולפי (Leiden) suggests one of the copyists or his predecessors miscopied whatever the original text read, most likely the negation in Paris. The fevers do not have to exhibit the signs of pestilential fevers in order for them to be compound humoral-pestilential types.

30 Emending "most of the heart" (רוב הלב) to "heart spirit" (רוח הלב) as in Leiden.

31 Emending ונתחלק to Paris's ונתלקח.

32 This is the opposite of what seems to be meant in Leiden.

33 שעול ורמ"ד—adopting Lola Ferre's suggestion of "tos y rheume"; see the note in Leiden.

34 "Their" refers to the humours' proportions.

35 Emending איור to אויר.

are altered to putrefied heat and moisture in a poisonous quality. But you should know that the pains and loss of strength at the onset of the sickness in pestilential fevers are more continuous and stronger than for humoral fevers [that derive] from breathing the putrefied air that is their unique, consistent cause.

CHAPTER: On the regimen for people with pestilence and the regimen for unadulterated pestilential fevers

THE REGIMEN for pestilential fevers, thus for those that occurred due to putrefaction and corruption of the air, putrefaction of the heart spirit [but] not the humours. When you realize that the air is putrefied **[fol. 139a]** and that the fevers are pestilential [according] to the signs we have mentioned, attend to correcting the air and people's regimen with things that remove the putrefaction. That means to leave the putrefied areas that are corrupting the air if the putrefied things are among the terrestrial causes we have indicated and to correct the putrefied air with fumigations and sprays from things that are cold, dry, and fragrant, with some drugs that have putrefaction-removing properties, rendering the air quality impervious to putrefaction so that the terrestrial cause of putrefaction from the regions causing the corruption makes no impression on the air. Even if the causes are celestial, these fumigations will prevent them. Know that the air is impressed when there is a planetary flux so that the malignant planet makes an impression on the local people who are predisposed by nature to receive it, the ones whose complexion diverges antithetically from that flux. Were it not for this, all the people exposed to[36] pestilential air would be acted upon to get pestilential sicknesses from which they would die or recover. But that is not what happens. Rather, some sicken and some do not, and the reason is whether or not they are predisposed to receive that flux. Therefore, the air should be corrected with things that give the air a quality opposing[37] the putrefaction and from the best things they can do for putrefied air that is pestilential according to the regimens for health for treating these fevers, treating people with dietary regimens and scents whose fumigation makes an impression on the humours and spirits to make them opposed and antithetical to the putrefaction, until they prevent or limit their receiving an impression from the corrupting air. This is when they burn fragrant wood and multiply bonfires in pestilential

---

36 Lit., "standing in."

37 Opposing, or counteracting.

places, especially myrtle trees, *ras marin*,[38] foxtail lily,[39] and citron, the herb hyssop and the other fragrant trees that counteract the putrefaction with the fragrance of their smoke [**fol. 139b**] and that destroy the putrefaction of the air. People should scent their clothing [by] dipping it in vinegar, and smell citron leaves and *serpoll*.[40] They should sprinkle the area with water and vinegar steeped with crushed sandalwood, roses, and myrtle, ten parts each with one part frankincense; citron leaves, *serpoll* leaves—an oz., two parts each; and it should be sprinkled where they are exposed,[41] and curtains soaked in these waters should be spread [across] the windows and the shutters locked. [This][42] will destroy the vapours from high in the pestilential air; then they will descend to the stony places, the thresholds and the stone-tiled houses [that have been] sprinkled with this—[do this] especially when it is time to sleep because the faculties are dormant and will not oppose the bad qualities that are inhaled as they would when they are wakened. For this reason, you would prevent sleep in those bitten by poisonous creatures, and those who have poisonous apostemes, those who are choking[43] and at the onset of the fever season. Their meals should have chicken and rooster, goat, suckling calves, and various types of small land and wild fowl, roasted in fire or in soup and vinegar and pomegranate juice, unripe wine, lemon juice, and citron vinegar. They should not eat much lamb, and those who eat pork should avoid[44] it and be cautious with organ meat. They should also avoid eating fish except the red rock fish with scales. How it should be eaten: fried[45] with vinegar, hyssop, a little onion, and Ceylonese cinnamon. They should avoid waterfowl and the spices they eat should mostly be sandalwood and Ceylonese cinnamon. They should avoid eating sweet fruits, especially moist dates and over-ripe [things] like squash and watermelon. They can eat any soured, unripe fruit, which is tightening and

38 Rosemary?

39 עריר. It appears in online searches as עריר לבנון, or *Eremurus* in the Asphodelaceae family, colloquially known in English as foxtail lily or desert candle.

40 The copyist transliterates the Romance *serpoll*. Leiden uses the Arabic *nimās*, then glosses with the Romance term. It is a type of wild thyme.

41 See note 36 above. Literally, in the place where they stand or are standing.

42 Lit., "it."

43 Presumably referring to a disease that makes it hard to breathe or swallow (like diphtheria or pneumonia).

44 "Avoid"—guard against. I use "avoid" in the following passages for וישמרו מ- except several lines below where a potion "guards against" corrupt spirit.

45 Or stewed?

astringent, like pomegranates, sour apples of moderate scent, black plums and plums,[46] stewed [fruits] **[fol.140a]** and apricots steeped in wine, and let them drink scented wine, appropriately mixed, and they should avoid milk and cheese. Let them begin their meal with a little onion with vinegar. Every morning, these people should drink fine white wine followed by a lemon electuary—1/2 scruple, which is ten grains of wheat—with *sigillata*. Alternatively, let them drink this potion: DRUG: citron peel, fresh garden wormwood, hyssop, myrtle—an ounce each. Ceylon cinnamon, sandalwood—½ oz. each. Armenian bole, *sigillata*—1 dram each. Sugar—3 litras. Rose water—½ litra. Let him make [this into] a potion; it will remove putrefaction, greatly strengthen the faculties, and clarify[47] the spirits. They should concoct another drink after refining pure, pulverized, crystal—2 drams, or clear [pome]granates pulverized and wrapped in a silk cloth or red silk.[48] They should always be kept in a storage jar; they will guard against corrupted scents. They should evacuate the humoral excess from people. If there is a plethora in the blood, they should be bled, and if there is an increase in one of the humours, they should be evacuated appropriately for fear of the putrefaction of the air being taken up in the superfluities in the humours and the spirits [quickly?] to the moisture deriving from them to oppose putrefactions.[49] DESCRIPTION: Smelling apple: DRUG: 3 types of sandalwood. Cinnamon, balsam—a dram each. Frankincense—½ oz. Camphor, myrrh—5 gr. each. Sulphur wort—3 drams. Ceylon cinnamon—3 drams. Sandalwood, muscatel[50]—a simple weight. BLHAN[51]—a dram. Lycium,[52]

---

46 Black plums—פרונש שחורות and plums—אגסים. Perhaps black and red plums?

47 יזהיר—lit., brighten.

48 In Leiden, fol. 119b, a white or red silk cloth.

49 Compare Leiden, fol. 119a, where the prose is even more convoluted. I'm not sure how to translate either version coherently, but Caslari indicates elsewhere that the danger in a humoral excess that has become putrefied (corrupted) is that it will pass to the spirits, ultimately reaching the heart. Something of the sort must be intended here.

50 Related to sandalwood. See glossary in *Tratado sobre la peste*, ed. Romeu Ferré. "Muscatelinos," a third variety of sandalwood (red, white, muscatel).

51 Or KLHAN?

52 Colloquially, box-thorn, also goji, which I think more likely here. McVaugh, Bos, and Shatzmiller, *The Regimen sanitatus of "Avenzoar,"* 145, section 3. According to Maimonides, it is dry and cleansing. See Gerrit Bos and Y. Tzvi Langermann, *Maimonides: On Rules Regarding the Practical Part of the Medical Art* (Provo: Brigham Young University Press, 2014), 238, no. 195, citing Book 4.5 of the Ibn Tibbon translation. Maimonides also describes "Indian lycium," כולאן הינדי, see Rosner,

lapadum[53]—a dram each; "white" mastic[54]—a dram. It can be compounded and made into a preserve[55] to be fumigated at night with the house closed; sprinkle with the above-mentioned water while fumigating.

CHAPTER: The regimen for those afflicted with an unadulterated pestilential fever.[56]

The regimen: Remove him from that air if possible, and if not, correct the air in the way [**fol. 140b**] we have mentioned. Turn to strengthening the heart with all might by means of food and therapeutic things, also with chickens roasted in sour things, lentil soup and white foods in lemon juice, and they should limit their [consumption of] almonds and flour, and drink white fragrant wine that is a little unripe,[57] pomegranate juice and citron vinegar steeped with *terra sigillata* and Armenian bole. He should eat sour fruit and specifically, moderately sweet pomegranates and apples, and particularly pomegranates and temperately fragrant apples, and white plums[58] that have ripened on the tree and whose color is like the colour of dark aubergines. He should eat horse radish with vinegar and also a compound of rose juice and a compound of lemon juice; let him smell sandalwood, myrtle and rose water steeped with camphor and saffron have been seeped—10 grains each;[59] frankincense—½ dr.; cinnamon, balsam—a dr.; fresh, crushed myrtle—an oz.; rose water—an oz. This should be boiled and placed in a silver vessel or

---

Moses Maimonides' Glossary of Drug Names, Book 6, section 7, and no. 123. The term also appears in Gerrit Bos and M. McVaugh, eds., *Maimonides: On Poisons and the Protection against Lethal Drugs* (Provo: Brigham Young University Press, 2009), 24, entry 64.

53 *Tratado sobre la peste*, ed. Romeu Ferré, p. 147, entry "Labdane." "Labdane: substancia resinosa que fluye de las hojas del arbusto llamado Cistus labdonifera Cretica." It is used in fumigations.

54 *'ilk*—mastic. *Ibn Janah*, eds., Bos et al., vol. 2, entry 715, pp. 864–65. Ibn Janah's entry is for "Nabatean mastic," so this is another variety. I am reading "albinum" as "white."

55 McVaugh, Bos, and Shatzmiller, *The Regimen sanitatus of "Avenzoar,"* 169 Eng., 144 Heb. Lola Ferre suggests a type of marinade in vinegar and vegetables ("escabeche"); email January 18, 2025.

56 Emending אויר (air) to דבר (pestilence), although, as the following sentence attests, "air" may have been somewhere in the original phrasing, perhaps "an unadulterated pestilential fever in the air?"

57 Or "weak."

58 Here, פרונש.

59 Leiden fol. 120a calls for one grain each. A "grain" typically meant a barley grain. Paris seems more reasonable.

a glass vessel in which white silk cloths are dipped and placed on the face, hands and nose. Make compresses for the heart from white or red silk cloths dipped in rose water with a little wine, apple juice, and a little vinegar; limit his sleep.

Evacuation of any sort is inappropriate, especially with a purgative, so that you do not evacuate the spirit that dissolves[60] and dissipates with evacuation, especially in turbulent air. And with this fever, an increase in humour does not require evacuation because what is good and necessary for the body would be evacuated along with the spirit. Moreover, most purgatives contain something poisonous and contrary to a healthy complexion and to the heart's faculties. In no case let blood for this fever, but if it is necessary he should be bled from the other side[61] after due consideration of timing. So, too, if an emetic is necessary just to eliminate excess [feces], they should do it after due consideration. Then he should drink this potion:

DRUG:
ASITOTA[62]—one litra; MeSYNA—an oz.; sandalwood and rose water [**fol. 141a**]—a half litra each; fresh or dried violets stripped of their pricks[63]—¼ litra; pomegranate juice—¼ litra; lemon juice—an oz.; juice of myrtle leaves—1 ½ oz.; sugar—3 litras. From this make a potion steeped with pure crystals and clear ruby,[64] pulverized and bound in a silk cloth, 10 grains each. He should drink from this as he wants. The sandalwood, violets and ASTOSA should be steeped, ground, for a day and night in the above-mentioned juices, then make the potion.

---

60 Emending as per Leiden fol. 120a, which has נתך (dissipates or dissolves) instead of Paris's נתק (separates).

61 Bleeding from the "other side" is called revulsion; bleeding from the same side as the affected site is called derivation. See Gil-Sotres, "Derivation and Revulsion;" Marganne, "Sur l'origine hippocratique des concepts de révulsion"; Voigts and McVaugh, "A Latin Technical Phlebotomy."

62 See a few lines below, ASTOSA, which must refer to the same plant, possibly related to *acetosella* (Lat.), *acetosella* (Cast.) or *ashtiyāllah* in "Spanish," and *rībās* in Arabic. According to Rosner, the Arabic term describes rhubarb-currant but the Spanish/Castillian refers to the (also sour) sorrel family. Rosner, *Maimonides' Glossary of Drug Names*, 246, no. 350.

63 See the introduction and the relevant note in Leiden: I think Caslari refers to garbling the dried violets but does not have a Hebrew word to describe "garbling," the process of stripping the dried flowers from the prickly stems.

64 Or another red stone like garnet or coral?

Chapter: *The regimen for those afflicted with humoral-pestilential fevers*

KNOW that there is no distinction in the regimen for those afflicted with the other fevers, the fainting, humoral, sanguine, choleric or phlegmatic, simple or compound, except that the sanguine should be bled, and those who have choleric and phlegmatic [fevers] should be purged; the humoral fevers should be treated with foods and medicines with care to the conditions of each. The humoral-pestilential fevers should be treated with the regimen for non-pestilential humoral fevers except that with humoral-pestilential fevers, attention to strengthening the heart must be greater than with non-pestilential [fevers], and he should attend to nourishing him more than he would for non-pestilential patients with foods suitable for fever and for the heart—even sometimes [with foods] that are not appropriate for fever but that taste better and are craved by the patient.

We already know that the faculties are strengthened[65] in the evening, so this should surely be done with supervision and much oversight. It is appropriate to feed him the meat that is suitable for him and to give him fragrant wine to drink that is well mixed, for the need for oversight is greater than it is for the humour, spirit and faculty.

Let the physician study the regimen for those afflicted with humoral [fevers] and treat them accordingly, turning to oversee the above-mentioned regimen for pestilential [fevers] for correcting the air. *Finished and Completed Praise to the Eternal God.*

65 Alternatively, "are retentive?"

GLOSSARY

HEBREW TO ENGLISH

Leiden = Leiden, MS or. 4778, and Paris = Paris, MS héb. 1191

אגס—plum (distinguished from פרונש, פרוניש, see below) (Paris 139b)
אוק', אונק', אוקייה, אונקייה—ounce
אופי—opium (Leiden 123a)
אותות—signs (of disease)
אותות מקדימות—prognosticating signs
אותות משיגים—accompanying signs
איבר, אבר—member ("solid member," or organ), sometimes limb (Leiden 115b, 116a; Paris 134a, 136a)
איזוב—hyssop (Leiden 119ab; Paris 139b, 140a)
אילן—tree, sometimes but not exclusively oak, and sometimes referring to acorns, branch or bark (Leiden 116b, 119a; Paris 135b, 136ab, 139a)
אלבירגיניש—aubergines (eggplant) (Paris 140b)
אלישנדרי—ALYSNDRY (alissandre? Alexander?) (Leiden 123b)
אסטניסות, אסטוטוט—weakness (Leiden115b, Paris 134a)
אסטושא, אסיטושא—*see also* חמצאניות, sorrel (wild) (Paris 140b, 141a)
אפסנתין—wormwood (Leiden 119b, 123ab; Paris 140a)
אפרסק—apricot (Leiden 119b, 123b; Paris 140a)
ארסיי—poisonous, venomous
ארבאטור, עשב טור—yarbatora, yerba tura, herbe toris, colloquially sulphurwort or hog's fennel (Leiden 119b; Paris 140a)
אשפרגי—asparagus (Leiden 123a)
אשקרופול—scruple (a weight)
אתרוג—citron (Leiden 119ab, 120a, 122b; Paris 138ab, 140b)

באבונג—chamomile, Ar. *Babunāj* (Leiden 122ab)
בדולח—crystal (Leiden 120b; Paris 140a, 141a)
בוסר—unripe wine (בוסר ענבים, unripe grapes or grape wine, Leiden 119a, 122a)
בוראגש—borage (Leiden 122b)
בשם, בושם—balsam (Leiden 119b, 120a, Paris 140ab)
בעל יציאות רבות—someone who defecates excessively (Leiden 123a)

גדמות—leprosy with loss of facial features and extremities, Ar. *ĝudham* (Leiden 116b; Paris 136a)
גדר—definition, category (Leiden 115b, 121b; Paris 135a)
גדרי—Ar. *judarī*, smallpox (Leiden 121b)
גיונברי—ginger (Leiden 119a)
גלגל—orbit (Leiden 117a; Paris 136b)
גראנט, גראנדש—granate (Leiden 119b; Paris 140a)

DOI: 10.17302/dohf208510 © Arc Humanities Press, 2026

דבוק—conjunction (astrological) (Leiden 121b)
דיאמינטא—*diamente*, a mint compound (Leiden 123a)
דלועים—pumpkin (Leiden 122b)
דלקת—causon fever (Leiden 118a)
דמיית—sanguine (Leiden 116a; Paris 136a)
דפק—pulse (Leiden 116a, Paris 136a)
דרהם—drachmē, dram (a measure); abbreviated 'דר and ʒ (Leiden 119b and note 32, 120ab, 122b, 123a; Paris 140ab)
דרציני—Chinese cinnamon (Ar., Pers. *Dar sīnī*) (Leiden 119b; Paris 139b, 140a)

הדס—myrtle (Leiden 119ab, 120a, 122b, 123a; Paris 139ab, 140ab)
הכנה—susceptibility, receptiveness, predisposition (Leiden 119a; Paris 139a)
הוליד—generate (Leiden 116a; Paris 135b)
הנהגה—regimen (Leiden 115a and note 1, 115b, 116b, 120b, 122a, Paris 135a, 140a)
הפכי—opposite, opposing (*see also* חולק) (Leiden 119a; Paris 139a)
הפסד—corruption (Leiden 116b, 117a, 118ab, 121a; Paris 135b, 136ab, 137a, 138ab)
הקדמת הידיעה—prognostication (Leiden 117b; Paris 137b); also found as אותות מקדימות—prognosticating signs (Leiden 117b, 118a; Paris 137b, 138a)
הקיז—let blood; הקזה —bloodletting, phlebotomy (Leiden 115a, 120a , 121a, 122a; Paris 134b, 140b)
הרויח—relieved, brought relief (from constipation) (Leiden 122ab); *see also* התיר.
הרקה—evacuation (Leiden 120a, 121a; Paris 140b)
השפיע שפע—to influence; or to cause an effluvia/flux (astrol.) (Leiden 117a, 118b, 119a, 121b; Paris 136b, 139a)
התחלה—onset (first fever stage)
התיר—released, loosened (constipation) (Paris 135a), and *see* הרויח.
In the *hof'al* form, יותר (Leiden 122a)
התחלה—onset (of fever), *see also* תחילה (Leiden 115ab, 121a, 122ab; Paris 134b, 135a, 138b, 139b)
התפשטות—spread, transmission (contagion) (Leiden 115b, 116ab, 117a, 118ab, 121b; Paris 135b, 136a, 138b)

ויאולש, ויאוליש, ויולש, ויאולט—violet (Leiden 120b, 122a, 123ab; Paris 141a)
ורד—rose (usually as מי ורד—rose water) (Leiden 119ab, 120a, 122ab, 123ab; Paris 139b, 140ab)

זיעה—sweat (Leiden 115a, 121a, 123a; Paris 134b)
זלוף—spray, spraying (Paris 139ab)
זעפראן—saffron (Leiden 120a, 122b, 123a)
זרעון—chickpea (Leiden 122b, 123a)

חולק—opposing, counteracting (*see also* הפכי) (Leiden 119a; Paris 139a)
חום טבעי—natural heat (Leiden 117a; Paris 137a)
חומץ—vinegar (Leiden 119ab, 120a, 122b, 123a; Paris 139b, 140ab)
חוקן—emetic (Leiden 120a, 122a; Paris 140b)
חזרת—horseradish (Leiden 120a, 122b; Paris 140b)
חמצאניות, חמצאעת—perhaps sorrel, identified with אבוקדולה (Leiden 120ab, 123a)
חפיפה—rubbing, massage (Leiden 122a)
חצבה—Ar. *hasaba*, measles (Leiden 121b)

חרחור—thirsting fever (Leiden 116b)
חרצון—fruit pips (Leiden 121b)
חריצי מים—aquifers, B. Ketubot 79b, e.g., B. Shabbat 73b and Rashi on Josh.11:8 (Leiden 116b; Paris 136b)

טיט ארמיני—Armenian bole (Leiden 119b, 120a)
טיט חתום—*terra sigillata* (Leiden 119b, 120a; Paris 140ab)

יותר—*see* התיר.

כח זן—nutritive faculty (Leiden 116b, Paris 136a)
כח חיוני—vital force/faculty (Leiden 116b, Paris 136a)
כח מאוה—appetitive faculty (Leiden 116b, Paris 136a)
כח מנהיג—unificative faculty (Paris 137a)
כח מעכל—digestive faculty (Leiden 116b; Paris 136a)
כלאן—Indian lycium (Ar. *Khulaan hindi*) (Paris 140a, note 34)
כפירים, כפר, כפרים—camphor, Ar. *Kafūr* (Leiden 119b, 120a, 122b; Paris 140a)
כרוב—cabbage (Leiden 123b)
כרכום—curcumin (turmeric) (Leiden 122a; Paris 135b, 136b)

לבונה—frankincense (Leiden 119ab, 120a, 123b; Paris 139b, 140ab)
לבלב—corriola, corregiola, Sp. corregúela; colloquial name in English is bindweed. There are two varieties, *libleb kabīr* and *libleb sagīr* (Leiden 122a, 123a)
לגלוגית—(Leiden 122b, 123b); also spelled חלגלוגות. Ibn Wāfid, *On Simple Drugs*, includes a listing for חלילג, where it is identified with myrobalans and used as a purgative.
להקיז—to let blood (Leiden 115a, 120a , 121a, 122a; Paris 134b, 140b)
להריק—to evacuate (Leiden 120a, 121a; Paris 140b)
לופינש—lupin(s) (Leiden 123b)
ליחה, ליחות—humour, humours (Leiden 116ab, 117ab, 118a, 120ab, 121a; Paris 135b, 136ab, 137a, 138ab, 140b, 141a); ליחיית, ליחיות —humoral (Leiden 116a, 118ab, 120b; Paris 136a, 141a)
ליטר, ליטרא—litra (pl. 'ליטרים, ליטר) (Leiden 119b, 120ab, 122b, 123ab; Paris 140ab, 141a)
לימוניש, לימונש—lemon (Leiden 119ab, 120a, 123ab; Paris 139b, 140b)
ליצאום—lycium, boxwood (Paris 140a)
לפאס—lampaza, acedera, lapazuela, also acedera, Catalan arengada, collerosa etc., and *Rumex pulcher* for the scientific label. *See* Ferre, *Práctica de Johannes de Parma* (John of Parma), 67, לאפסה. This may be the herb colloquially called fiddle dock in English (Leiden 123a, as לפאס האגודה, perhaps a bundle or bunch of fiddle dock)
לפדנום—ladanum, Sp. Labadano, láudano, a compound including wine, opium, and saffron (Romeu Ferré 2024: 88, 108)
לשלשל—to purge (Leiden 120a, 122a; Paris 140b)

מוגמר—incense (Leiden 119b; Paris 140a)
מור—myrrh (Leiden 119b; Paris 140a)
מזג—complexion (humoral) (Leiden 117a, 118ab, 119a, 120ab; Paris 136b, 137a, 138b, 139a, 141a)
מזוקק—unadulterated, pure (Leiden 118b, 119b; Paris 138b, 140a)
מלונש—melon (Leiden 122b)

מלילוט—meliote (Leiden 122a)
ממוצע—moderate (Leiden 119b, 120a; Paris 139b, 140b)
מנא נאר—mana nār? Unidentified. (Leiden 122a)
מצוקה—pain (Leiden 115a, 116a, 118a, 122b; Paris 134b, 135b, 138ab)
מצטיק—mastic (Leiden 123ab); *see also* עלך
מרקואיל—*mercurialis annua*, annual mercury (Leiden 123a)
מקרה—symptom (Leiden 115a, 116b, 117ab, 118a, 120b, 122a; Paris 134b, 136a, 137ab, 138a)
מרחשת—fried? Or stewed? (Leiden 119b)
מררת פר—ox gall (Leiden 123b)
משיחה—ointment (Leiden 122b, 123ab)
משינה—perhaps iris (Leiden 120a)
משפטי הכוכבים—laws of astrology (astronomy) (Leiden 117ab, 121b; Paris 137ab)
משרת פשתן—where linen is soaked, *see* Mishnah Ber. 3:5 (Paris 135b)
מתפשט—transmissible (spreading, contagious) (Leiden 115b, 116ab; Paris 135b, 136b) (also התפשטות)

נדבי, הנדבי—endive (Leiden 123a)
נדבק—was in (astrological) conjunction (Leiden 121b)
נשדף—lit., blighted, but referring to someone with hectic fever (Leiden 116b; Paris 136a)
נתך—dissolves (Paris 138a)

סגולה—property, characteristic, attribute (Leiden 118ab, 121b; Paris 138a, 139a)
סומאק—sumac (Leiden 123a)
סיבה חמרית—material cause (Leiden 121a)
סינאמומי—cinnamon (Leiden 123b)
סינטוניקא—SYNTVNYQA ? (Leiden 123b)
סלעי האדום—red rock fish (Leiden 119b; Paris 139b)
סלקא—beet (Leiden 122a)
סנטוריאה—centaura (Leiden 123b)
סתר, לסתור—to destroy (Paris 139b)

עדשים—lentils (Leiden 120a, 122b; Paris 140b)
עונות הקדחת—stages or phases (lit., "seasons") of a fever (Leiden 119a; Paris 139b)
עלוף—fainting (Leiden 115b, Paris 134a); קדחת עלופית או עלפית—fainting fever (Leiden 120b, 121a; Paris 141a)
עלוקה—leech (Leiden 122a)
עלייה—increase (second fever stage) (Leiden 115b, 122b; Paris 135a)
עלך—mastic (Ar.) (Paris 140a)
עפץ—astringent (a drug quality) (Leiden 119b; Paris 139b)
עפש—putrefy (עיפוש—putrefaction); to putrefy—לעפש; used throughout.
ערבה—willow (Leiden 122a)
ערמון—chestnut (Leiden 121b)
ערער—possibly the plant עריר הלבנון, Eremurus, foxtail lily or desert candle (Paris 139a)
עשון—fumigation (Leiden 118b; Paris 139a)

פאפאויר—papaver (Leiden 123a)
פוטר—parsley (Leiden 122b)

פויליפודי—polipode (bisbeige) (Leiden 122a)
פום טירא—*fumus terre*, fumaria (Leiden 123a)
פופוליון—popolion? unidentified (Leiden 122b)
פורח—dissipates (Leiden 120a; Paris 140b)
פרונש, פרוניש, פירניש—plums (Leiden 119b, 122ab; Paris 139b, 140b)
פלגירה—FLGYRH? (Leiden 123b)
פרנשין, פרינישין—phrenitis (frenesie) (Leiden 115b; Paris 134a)

צבר—aloe (Leiden 123b)
צירפויל, צירפוייל—*serpoll* (also spelled שרפול), Arabic *nimās*, a type of wild thyme (Leiden 119b; Paris 139b)
צנדליש, צנדיל, צאנדיל—sandalwood (Leiden 119ab, 120ab, 122b, 123a; Paris 139b, 140ab)
צער—anguish, distress (Paris 137b)
קדחת—fever
אדומית—choleric fever (Leiden 115a, 118a, 120b; Paris 135a, 138b, 141a)
  בלתי פוסקת—continuous (lit., uninterrupted) fever (Leiden 115a, Paris 134b)
  דברית—pestilential fever (throughout both copies)
  לבנית—phlegmatic fever (Leiden 118a, 120b ; Paris 138b, 141a)
  ליחיית, לחיית—humoral fever (Leiden 118a, 120b; Paris 138a)
  מורכבת—compound fever (Leiden 120b; Paris 141a)
  מתמידית—continuous fever (*see also* תמידיית) (Leiden 115ab; Paris 134a)
  עלפית—fainting fever; *see* עלוף, עלפית
  פשוטה—simple fever (Leiden 120b, 121a; Paris 141a)

קובץ—tightening (a drug property) (Leiden 116b, 119a; Paris 139b)
קוהה, קוהא—sour, unripe (Leiden 119b, 120a; Paris 139b, 140b)
קושיש—QVSYS? (Leiden 122a)
קטור—fumigating, burning incense (Leiden 119b; Paris 139a, 140a); *see also* עשון
קיא—vomiting, vomit (להקיא) (Leiden 115ab, 121a, 122a; Paris 134b, 135a)
קנמון—cinnamon, also spelled סינאמומי (Leiden 119b, 120a, 123b; Paris 140ab)
קפילי ונירש—*Capillus veneris*, or maidenhead fern (Leiden 123a)
קרבים—entrails, hence organ meat (Paris 139b)
קרישוש—QRYSVS? (Leiden 123a)
קרישפיניל—QRYSPYNYL? (crespinal?) (Leiden 123b)
קרש—crumbles, disintegrates (Leiden 123a)

רבברביר—rhubarb (Leiden 122a)
רוח—spirit, pneuma (used throughout)
רושם—stamp, impression (Leiden 118b, 119a; Paris 135b,139a)
רימון, רמון—pomegranate (Leiden 119a, 122b, 123b; Paris 139b, 140b, 141a)
רוש מרין—rosemary? (Paris 139a)

שדפון—hectic fever; those with hectic fever—נשדפים (Leiden 116b; Paris 136b)
שווי—equilibrium (Leiden 117b; Paris 137b); equinox (Leiden 121b)
שלוק—scalded (Leiden 122a)
שלשל—to purge, evacuate (Leiden 120a, 122a; Paris 140b); שלשול—purging (Leiden 115a, 121a, 122a, 123a; Paris 134b, 138a)
שעוה—wax (Leiden 122b)
שקדים—almonds (Leiden 120a, 122b, 123ab; Paris 140b)

שקוי—dropsy (Leiden 121a)
שפרול—*see* צירפול, צירפויל; *serpoll*
שתן—urine (Leiden 115a, 116a, 117b; Paris 135ab, 136a, 137ab)
תגבורת ליחה—increase in a humour (Leiden 117ab, 118a, 120a, 121a; Paris 137ab, 140b)
תחילה—onset (of disease or fever) (Leiden 121a); *see* התחלה.
תולעת שני—red silk (Leiden 119b,120a; Paris 140ab)
תועלת כללית—common good (Leiden 115b; Paris 135a)
תות—mulberry (Leiden 122b)
תכלית—duration (third fever stage) (Leiden 117a; Paris 135a,137a)
תעורה—agitation, turbulence, wakefulness (Leiden 115a, 116a, 117b, 122b; Paris 135a, 136a, 137a)
תפוח להריח—smelling apple (a sachet) (Leiden 119b; Paris 140a).
תפוחים ריחניים—fragrant apples (Leiden 119b, 122b; Paris 140b)

GLOSSARY

ENGLISH TO HEBREW

acorn—אילן (Leiden 121b). *See also* "tree"
agitation (also turbulence, wakefulness)—תעורה (Leiden 115a, 116a, 117b, 122b; Paris 135a, 136a, 137a(
almonds—שקדים (Leiden 120a, 122b, 123ab; Paris 140b)
aloe—צבר (Leiden 123b)
ALYSNDRY (alissandre? Alexander?)—אלישנדרי (Leiden 123b)
anguish, distress—צער (Paris 137b)
apricot—אפרסק (Leiden 119b, 123b; Paris 140a)
aquifers—חריצי מים (Leiden 116b; Paris 136b)
Armenian bole—טיט ארמיני (Leiden 119b, 120a)
asparagus—אשפרגי (Leiden 123a)
astringent (drug quality)—עפץ (Leiden 119b; Paris 139b)
aubergine (eggplant)—אלבירגיניש (Paris 140b)

balsam—בשם, בושם (Leiden 119b, 120a, Paris 140ab)
beet—סלקא (Leiden 122a)
bleed, let blood—הקיז; bloodletting, phlebotomy—הקזה (Leiden 115a, 120a, 121a, 122a; Paris 134b, 140b)
borage—בוראגש (Leiden 122b)

camphor, Ar. *Kafūr* —כפירים, כפר, כפרים (Leiden 119b, 120a, 122b; Paris 140a)
Capillus veneris, or maidenhead fern—קפילי ונריש (Leiden 123a)
causon (fever type)—דלקת (Leiden 118a)
centaura—סנטוריאה (Leiden 123b)
chamomile (Ar. *Babūnāj*)—באבונג (Leiden 122ab)
chestnut—ערמון (Leiden 121b)
chickpea—זרעון (Leiden 122b, 123a)
cinnamon—קינמון, also סינאמומי (Leiden 119b, 120a, 123b; Paris 140ab)
citron—אתרוג (Leiden 119ab, 120a, 122b; Paris 138ab, 140b)
common good—תועלת כללית (Leiden 115b; Paris 135a)
complexion (humoral mix)—מזג (Leiden 117a, 118ab, 119a, 120ab; Paris 136b, 137a, 138b, 139a, 141a)
conjunction (astrological)—דבוק (Leiden 121b)
corriola, corregiola, Sp. Corregúela; colloquial English bindweed. There are two varieties, *libleb kabīr* and *libleb sagīr*—לבלב (Leiden 122a, 123a)
corruption (humoral)—הפסד (Leiden 116b, 117a, 118ab, 121a; Paris 135b, 136ab, 137a, 138ab)
curcumin (turmeric)—כרכום (Leiden 122a; Paris 135b, 136b)
crumbles, disintegrates—קרש (Leiden 123a)
crystal—בדולח (Leiden 120b; Paris 140a, 141a)

DOI: 10.17302/dohf208511 © Arc Humanities Press, 2026

definition, or category—גדר (Leiden 115b, 121b; Paris 135a)
destroy—סתר (לסתור) (Paris 139b)
diamente—דיאמינטא, a mint compound (Leiden 123a)
digestive faculty—כח מעכל (Leiden 116b; Paris 136a)
dissipates—פורח (Leiden 120a; Paris 140b)
dissolves—נתך (Paris 138a)
drachmē, dram (a measure)—דרהם, abbreviated דר' and ʒ (Leiden 119b and note 32, 120ab, 122b, 123a; Paris 140ab)
dropsy—שקוי (Leiden 121a)
duration (third fever stage)—תכלית (Leiden 117a; Paris 135a, 137a)

emetic—חוקן (Leiden 120a, 122a; Paris 140b)
endive—נדבי, הנדבי (Leiden 123a), an astringent
equilibrium—שווי (Leiden 117b; Paris 137b); *see also* equinox.
equinox—שווי (Leiden 121b)
Eremurus—see foxtail lily
evacuation—הרקה (Leiden 120a, 121a; Paris 140b)
excessive defecation—יציאות רבות (Leiden 123a); someone who defecates excessively—בעל יציאות רבות

fainting—עלוף (Leiden 115b, Paris 134a); fainting fever—קדחת עלופית או עלפית (Leiden 120b, 121a; Paris 141a)
fever—קדחת
  choleric fever—קדחת אדומית (Leiden 115a, 118a, 120b; Paris 135a, 138b, 141a)
  compound fever—קדחת מורכבת (Leiden 120b; Paris 141a)
  continuous fever—קדחת מתמידית, תמידיית (Leiden 115ab; Paris 134a)
  fainting fever—קדחת עלפית, עלופית. *See* עלוף, עלפית
  humoral fever—קדחת לחיית, ליחיית (Leiden 118a, 120b; Paris 138a)
  phlegmatic fever—קדחת לבנית (Leiden 118a, 120b; Paris 138b, 141a)
  simple fever—קדחת פשוטה (Leiden 120b, 121a; Paris 141a)
FLGYRH?—פלגירה (Leiden 123b)
foxtail lily—עריר הלבנון and possibly intended by Caslari's ערער; also known as desert candle, scientific name *Eremurus* (Paris 139a)
frankincense—לבונה (Leiden 119ab, 120a, 123b; Paris 139b, 140ab)
fried? (or stewed)—מרחשת (Leiden 119b)
fruit pips—חרצון (Leiden 121b)
fumigation—עשון (Leiden 118b; Paris 139a). *See also* קטור
fumigating (incense)—קטור; fumigation—הקטרה (Leiden 119b; Paris 139a, 140a)
Fumus terre (fumaria)—פום טירא (Leiden 123a)

generate—הוליד (Leiden 116a; Paris 135b)
ginger—גיונברי (Leiden 119a)
granate—גראנט, גראנדש (Leiden 119b; Paris 140a)

hectic fever—שדפון, someone afflicted with hectic fever—נשדף (Leiden 116b; Paris 136a); lit., blighted.
horseradish—חזרת (Leiden 120a, 122b; Paris 140b)

humour—ליחה (pl. ליחות) (Leiden 116ab, 117ab, 118a, 120ab, 121a; Paris 135b, 136ab, 137a, 138ab, 140b, 141a(; ליחיית, ליחיות—humoral (Leiden 116a, 118ab, 120b; Paris 136a, 141a)
hyssop—איזוב (Leiden 119ab; Paris 139b, 140a)

impression—*see* stamp
incense—מוגמר (Leiden 119b; Paris 140a)
increase (fever stage)—עלייה (Leiden 115b, 122b; Paris 135a)
increase (in a humour)—תגבורת ליחה (Leiden 117ab, 118a, 120a, 121a; Paris 137ab, 140b)
Indian lycium (Ar. Khulaan hindi)—כלאן, כלהאן (Paris 140a, note 34)
influence (vt.) or cause an effluvia (astrol.)—השפיע שפע (Leiden 117a, 118b, 119a, 121b; Paris 136b, 139a)
iris?—משינה (Leiden 120a)

lampaza, acedera, lapazuela, also acedera, Catalan arengada, collerosa, etc.—לפאס, in Ferre, *Práctica de Johannes de Parma*, 67, לאפסה. The scientific name is *Rumex pulcher*, and the herb may be what is colloquially called fiddledock in English (Leiden 123a, where it appears as לפאס האגודה, perhaps a bundle or bunch of fiddledock).
laws of astrology/astronomy—משפטי הכוכבים (Leiden 117ab, 121b; Paris 137ab)
leprosy with loss of facial features and extremities (Ar. *Ĝudham*)—גדמות (Leiden 116b; Paris 136a)
lemon—לימוניש, לימונש (Leiden 119ab, 120a, 123ab; Paris 139b, 140b)
lentils—עדשים (Leiden 120a, 122b; Paris 140b)
litra—ליטרא ליטר, ליט', (pl., ליטרי' ליטרים) (Leiden 119b, 120ab, 122b, 123ab; Paris 140ab, 141a)
lupin(s)—לופינש (Leiden 123b)
lycium, boxwood—ליצאום (Paris 140a)

Mana nār? MN' N'R—מנא נאר Unidentified (Leiden 122a)
mastic—מצטיק (Leiden 123ab); also Arabic עלך (Paris 140a)
material cause—סיבה חמרית (Leiden 121a)
measles—חצבה, Ar. *hasaba* (Leiden 121b)
meliote—מלילוט (Leiden 122a)
melon—מלונש (Leiden 122b)
member (or limb)—איבר, אבר (Leiden 115b, 116a; Paris 134a, 136a)
Mercurialis annua (annual mercury)—מרקואיל (Leiden 123a)
moderate—ממוצע (Leiden 119b, 120a; Paris 139b, 140b)
mulberry—תות (Leiden 122b)
myrobalans—Possibly indicated by the terms לגולוגית, חלוגלוגות. Ibn Wāfid's compendium of simple drugs lists חלילג, which he identified with myrobalans; a purgative.
myrtle—הדס (Leiden 119ab, 120a, 122b, 123a; Paris 139ab, 140ab)

natural heat—חום טבעי (Leiden 117a; Paris 137a)

ointment—משיחה (Leiden 122b, 123ab)
onset (fever stage)—התחלה (Leiden 115ab, 119a, 121a, 122ab; Paris 134b, 135ab); *see also* תחילה

opium—אופי (Leiden 123a)
opposing, counteracting—חולק (Leiden 119a; Paris 139a); *see also* הפכי
opposite, opposing—הפכי (Leiden 119a; Paris 139a)
orbit, revolution—גלגל (Leiden 117a; Paris 136b)
organ meat (entrails)—קרבים (Paris 139b)
ounce—אוק׳, אונק׳, אוקייה, אונקייה
ox gall—מררת פר (Leiden 119b)

pain—מצוקה (Leiden 115a, 116a, 118a, 122b; Paris 134b, 135b, 138ab)
papaver—פאפאויר (Leiden 123a)
parsley—פוטר (Leiden 122b)
phrenitis (frenesie)—פרנשין, פרינישין (Leiden 115b; Paris 134a)
plum—אגס (Paris 139b)
plum—פרונש, פרוניש, פירניש (Leiden 119b, 122ab; Paris 139b,140b)
poisonous (venomous)—ארסיי
polipode (bisbeige)—פויליפודי (Leiden 122a)
pomegranate—רימון, רמון (Leiden 119a, 122b, 123b; Paris 139b, 140b, 141a)
POPOLYON (?)—פופוליון (Leiden 122b)
prognostication—הקדמת הידיעה (Leiden 117b; Paris 137b), also found as אותות מקדימות—prognosticating signs (Leiden 117b, 118a; Paris 137b, 138a)
property (characteristic, attribute)—סגולה (Leiden 118ab, 121b; Paris 138a, 139a)
pulse—דפק (Leiden 116a; Paris 136a)
pumpkins—דלועים (Leiden 122b, 123a)
purge, evacuate—לשלשל (Leiden 120a, 122a; Paris 140b).
purging—שלשול (Leiden 115a, 121a, 122a, 123a; Paris 134b, 138a)
putrefaction—עפוש (to putrefy: לעפש), used throughout both MSS

QRYSPYNYL?—קרישפיניל (crespinal?) (Leiden 123b)
QRYSVS?—קרישוש (Leiden 123a)
QVSYS ?—קושיש (Leiden 122a)

red rock fish—סלעי האדום (Leiden119b; Paris 139b)
red silk—תולעת שני (Leiden 119b,120a; Paris 140ab)
regimen—הנהגה (Leiden 115a and note 1, 115b, 116b, 120b, 122a; Paris 135a, 140a)
released, loosened (constipation)—התיר (Paris 135a); *see also* הרויח
relieved, brought relief (from constipation)—הרויח (Leiden 122ab, 123a); *see also* התיר
rhubarb—רבברביר (Leiden 122a)
rose—ורד, usually as rose water—מי ורד (Leiden 119ab, 120a, 122ab, 123ab; Paris 139b, 140ab)
rosemary?—רוש מרין (Paris 139a)
rubbing, massage—חפיפה (Leiden 122a)

saffron—זעפראן (Leiden 120a, 122b, 123a)
sandalwood—צאנדיל צנדליש, צנדיל, (Leiden 119ab, 120ab, 122b, 123a; Paris 139b, 140ab)
sanguine—דמיית (Leiden 116a; Paris 136a)
scalded—שלוק (Leiden 122a)
scruple (a weight measure)—אשקרופול
serpoll—צירפוייל, צירפויל and שרפול; Arabic *nimās*, a type of wild thyme (Leiden 119b; Paris 139b)

signs (of disease)—אותות
    accompanying signs—אותות משיגות
prognosticating signs—אותות מקדימות
smallpox—Ar. *judarī*, גדרי (Leiden 121b)
smelling apple (a sachet)—תפוח להריח (Leiden 119b; Paris 140a). תפוחים ריחניים—fragrant apples (Leiden 119b, 122b; Paris 140b)
sorrel (wild)—אסטושא, אסיטושא; *see also* חמצאניות (Paris 140b, 141a)
sorrel?—חמצאניות, חמצאעת, identified with אבוקדולה (Leiden 120ab, 123a)
sour, unripe—קוהה, קוהא (Leiden 119b, 120a; Paris 139b, 140b)
spirit, pneuma—רוח (used throughout)
spray, spraying—זלוף (Paris 139ab(
spread, transmission (contagion)—התפשטות (Leiden 115b, 116ab, 117a, 118ab, 121b; Paris 135b, 136a, 138b)
stages or phases (lit., "seasons") of the fever—עונות הקדחת (Leiden 119a; Paris 139b)
stamp, impression—רושם (Leiden 118b, 119a; Paris135b, 139a)
stewed? (or fried)—מרחשת (Leiden 119b)
sulphur wort—ארבאטור, עשב טור (*see also* yarbatora, also called yerba tura, herbe toris, and hog's fennel) (Leiden 119b; Paris 140a)
sumac—סומאק (Leiden 123a)
susceptibility, receptiveness, predisposition—הכנה (Leiden 119a; Paris 139a)
sweat—זיעה (Leiden 115a, 121a, 123a; Paris 134b)
symptom—מקרה (Leiden 115a, 116b, 117ab, 118a, 120b, 122a; Paris 134b, 136a, 137ab, 138a)
SYNTVNYQA?—סינטוניקא (Leiden 123b)

Terra sigillata—טיט חתום (Leiden 119b, 120a; Paris 140ab)
thirsting fever—חרחור (Leiden 116b)
tightening (a drug property)—קובץ (Leiden 116b, 119a; Paris 139b)
transmissible (contagious, spreading)—מתפשט (Leiden 115b, 116ab; Paris 135b, 136b) (also התפשטות)
tree, sometimes specifically oak—אילן (Leiden 116b, 119a; Paris 135b, 136ab, 139a)

unadulterated, pure—מזוקק (Leiden 118b, 119b; Paris 138b, 140a)
unificative faculty—כח מנהיג (Paris 137a)
unripe wine—בוסר; unripe grapes or grape wine—בוסר ענבים (Leiden 119a, 122a)
urine—שתן (Leiden 115a, 116a, 117b, Paris 135ab, 136a, 137ab)

vinegar—חומץ (Leiden 119ab, 120a, 122b, 123a; Paris 139b, 140ab)
violet—ויאולש, ויאוליש, ויולש, ויאולט (Leiden 120b, 122a, 123ab; Paris 141a)
vomiting, vomit—קיא (להקיא) (Leiden 115ab, 121a, 122a; Paris 134b, 135a)

wax—שעווה (Leiden 122b)
weakness—אסטניסות, אסטוטוט (Leiden 115b, Paris 134a)
willow—ערבה (Leiden 122a)
wormwood—אפסנתין (Leiden 119b, 123ab; Paris 140a)

yarbatora—ארבאטור,עשב טור (*see* sulphur wort; yerba tura, herbe toris, and hog's fennel) (Leiden 119b; Paris 140a)

SELECT BIBLIOGRAPHY

Aberth, John. *Doctoring the Black Death: Medieval Europe's Medical Response to Plague*. Lanham: Rowman & Littlefield, 2021.

Andrades Valtueña, Aida, et al. "The Stone Age Plague and its Persistence in Eurasia." *Current Biology* 27 (2017): 3683–89.

Armstrong-Partida, Michele. *Defiant Priests: Domestic Unions, Violence and Clerical Masculinity in Fourteenth-Century Catalunya*. Ithaca: Cornell University Press, 2017.

Arrizabalaga, Jon. "Facing the Black Death: Perceptions and Reactions of University Medical Practitioners." In *Practical Medicine from Salerno to the Black Death*, edited by Luis García Ballester, Roger French, Jon Arrizabalaga and Andrew Cunningham, 237–88. Cambridge: Cambridge University Press, 1994.

Ballan, Mohamad. "Borderland Anxieties: Lisān al-Dīn ibn al-Khaṭīb and the Politics of Genealogy in Late Medieval Granada." *Speculum* 98, no. 2 (2023): 447–95.

Barkai, Ron. "Jewish Treatises on the Black Death, 1300–1500: A Preliminary Study." In *Medicine from the Black Death to the French Disease*, edited by Roger French, Jon Arrizabalaga, Andrew Cunningham and Luis García Ballester, 6–25. Aldershot: Ashgate, 1998.

Barker, Hannah. "Laying the Corpses to Rest: Grain, Embargoes, and *Yersinia pestis* in the Black Sea, 1346–48." *Speculum* 96, no. 1 (2021): 97–126.

Barzilay, Tzafrir. "The Black Death in Aragon: Notes on a Jewish Chronicle" [in Hebrew]. *Hayo Haya* 8 (2011): 53–71.

——. *Poisoned Wells: Accusations, Persecution and Minorities in Medieval Europe, 1321–1422*. Philadelphia: University of Pennsylvania Press, 2022.

Beltrán de Heredia Bercero, Julie, and I. Gibrat Pineda. "El primer testimoni arqueològic de la Pesta Negra a Barcelona: La fossa comuna de la Basília dels Sants Màrtirs Just i Pastor." *Quarhis* 2, no. 10 (2014): 164–75.

Benedictow, Ole. *The Black Death 1346–1353: The Complete History*. Woodridge: Boydell and Brewer, 2004.

Benito i Monclús, Pere, and Antoni Riera i Melis, eds. *Guerra y carestía en la Europa medieval*. Lleida: Milenia, 2014.

Bensch, Stephen P. "A Baronial Aljama: The Jews of Empúries in the Thirteenth Century." *Jewish History* 22, nos. 1–2 (2008): 19–51.

Bos, Gerrit. *A Concise Dictionary of Novel Medical and General Hebrew Terminology from the Middle Ages*. Leiden: Brill, 2019.

——. *Ibn al-Jazzār on Fevers: The Original Arabic Text with an English Translation, Introduction, and Commentary*. London: Kegan Paul, 2000.

——. *Novel Medical and General Hebrew Terminology from the Thirteenth Century*. Supplement 27, *Journal of Semitic Studies*. Oxford: Oxford University Press, 2011.

Bos, Gerrit, et al., eds. *Marwān ibn Janāh: On the Nomenclature of Medicinal Drugs (Kitāb al-Talkhīs)*. Leiden: Brill, 2020.

Bos, Gerrit, and Y. Tzvi Langermann, eds. *Maimonides: On Rules Regarding the Practical Part of the Medical Art*. Provo: Brigham Young University Press, 2014.

Bos, Gerrit, and Michael McVaugh. *Maimonides: On Poisons and the Protection against Lethal Drugs*. Provo: Brigham Young University Press, 2009.

DOI: 10.17302/dohf208512

Bos, Gerrit, and Guido Mensching. "The Black Death in Hebrew Literature: Abraham Ben Solomon Hen's *Tractatulus de Pestilentia*." *Jewish Studies Quarterly* 18 (2011): 32–63.

Bos, Gerrit, Charles Burnett, and Y. Tzvi Langermann. *Hebrew Medical Astrology: David Ben Yom Tov, Kelal Qatan, Original Hebrew Text, Medieval Latin Translation, Modern English Translation*. Philadelphia: American Philosophical Society, 2005.

Bos, Gerrit, Michael McVaugh, and Joseph Shatzmiller. *Transmitting a Text through Three Languages: The Future History of Galen's Peri Anomalou Dyskrasias*. Philadelphia: Transactions of the American Philosophical Society, 2014. New series 104, no. 5: 1–168.

Bos, Kirsten I., Verena Schuenemann, G. Brian Golding, et al. "A Draft Genome of *Yersinia pestis* from Victims of the Black Death." *Nature* 478 (2011): 506–10.

Brain, Peter. *Galen on Bloodletting*. Cambridge: Cambridge University Press, 2009.

Burridge, Claire. *Carolingian Medical Knowledge and Practice c. 775–900: New Approaches to Recipe Literature*. Leiden: Brill, 2024.

Callico, Jaume Sobreques. "La Pesta Negra en la península ibérica." *Anuario de estudios medievales* 7 (1970–1971): 67–102.

Carmichael, Ann. *Plague and the Poor in Renaissance Florence*. Cambridge: Cambridge University Press, 1986.

——. "Universal and Particular: The Language of Plague 1348–1500." *Medical History Supplement* 27 (2008): 17–52.

Carpentieri, Nicola, Alexander Fidora, and Isaac Lampurlanés. "Avicena y Gerardo de Cremona sobre la frenitis: Una comparación entre al-Qānūn fī ṭ-Ṭibb y su traducción latina." *Al-Qanṭara* 39, no. 2 (2018): 293–320.

Carpentieri, Nicola, and Taro Mimura. "Arabic Commentaries on the Hippocratic Aphorisms, vi.11: A Medieval Medical Debate on Phrenitis." *Oriens* 45, nos. 1–2 (2017): 176–202.

Chase, Melissa. "Fevers, Poisons and Apostemes: Authority and Experience in Montpellier Plague Treatises." *Annals of the New York Academy of Sciences* 441 (1985): 153–69.

Chouin, Gerard. "Reflections on Plague in African History (14th–19th century)." *Afriques* 9 (September 2018), https://doi.org/10.4000/afriques.2228.

Cohen Hanegbi, Na'ama. "Transmitting Medicine Across Religions: Jean of Avignon's Hebrew Translation of the *Lilium Medicine*." In *Latin-into-Hebrew: Texts and Studies*, edited by Resianne Fontaine and Gad Freudenthal, 1:121–45. Leiden: Brill, 2013.

Colet, Anna, Josep Xavier Muntané, Jordi Ruiz Ventura, Oriol Saula, M. Eulàlia Subirà de Galdàcano, and Clara Jáuregui. "The Black Death and its Consequences for the Jewish Community in Tàrrega: Lessons from History and Archeology." In *Pandemic Disease in the Medieval World*, edited by Monica Green, special issue of *The Medieval Globe* 1 (2014): 63–96.

Collar, Anna, ed. *Networks and the Spread of Ideas in the Past: Strong Ties, Innovation, and Knowledge Exchange*. New York: Routledge, 2022.

Davidson, Israel, *Shalosh halatzot* [Three Parodies]. New York: n.p., 1904.

Demaitre, Luke. "The Art and Science of Prognostication in Early University Medicine." *Bulletin of the History of Medicine* 77, no. 4 (2003): 765–88.

——. *Doctor Bernard de Gordon, Professor and Practitioner*. Toronto: Pontifical Institute of Mediaeval Studies, 1980.

——. *Medieval Medicine: The Art of Healing, from Head to Toe*. Santa Barbara: Praeger/ABC-CLIO, 2013.

DeVos, Paula. "European Materia Medica in Historical Texts: Longevity of a Tradition and Implications for Future Use." *Journal of Ethnopharmacology* 132, no. 1 (2010): 1–46.

DeWitte, Sharon, Julia Beaumont, Brittany S. Walter, Jacqueline R. Towers, and Emily J. Brennan. "Childhood Nutritional Stress and Later-Life Health Outcomes in Medieval England: Evidence from Incremental Dentine Analysis." *Science Advances* (July 30, 2025): https://doi.10.1126/sciadv.adw7076.

Di Segni, Diana. "Gentile da Foligno's *Consilium contra Pestilantium* and its Hebrew Translation," *Quaderni di Noctua* 7 (2024): 218–63.

——. "Latin-into-Hebrew Treatises on the Black Death." In *Epidemics and Pandemics*, edited by Michele Nicoletti and Alessandro Palazzo, 105–30. Turnhout: Brepols, 2024.

Dols, Michael, *The Black Death in the Midde East*. Princeton: Princeton University Press, 1977.

Einbinder, Susan L. *After the Black Death: Plague and Commemoration Among Iberian Jews*. Philadelphia: University of Pennsylvania Press, 2018.

——. "Drought and Plague in Fifteenth-century Algiers: The Hymns of R. Simon ben Zemah Duran." *Medieval Encounters* (2026). Forthcoming.

——. *No Place of Rest: Jewish Literature, Expulsion, and the Memory of Medieval France*. Philadelphia: University of Pennsylvania Press, 2008.

Einbinder, Susan L., and Michael McVaugh. "Latin into Hebrew—Twice Over! Presenting Latin Scholastic Medicine to a Jewish Audience." In *Latin into Hebrew: Texts and Studies*, edited by Resianne Fontaine and Gad Freudenthal, vol. 1, 31–44 and appendix, 455–68. 2 vols. Leiden: Brill, 2013.

Emery, Richard. "The Black Death in Perpignan." *Speculum* 42, no. 4 (1967): 611–23.

Fancy, Nahyan. "Medical Commentaries: A Preliminary Examination." *Oriens* 41 (2013): 525–45.

——. *Science and Religion in Mamluk Egypt: Ibn al-Nafīs, Pulmonary Transit and Bodily Resurrection*. London: Routledge, 2013.

Fancy, Nahyan, and Monica H. Green, "Plague and the Fall of Baghdad (1258)." *Medical History* 65, no. 2 (2021): 155–77.

Faraudo de Saint-Germain, Luis. *El "Libre de les medicines particulars": Version catalana trescentista del texto árabe del Tratado de los medicamentos simples de Ibn Wáfid, autor médico toledano del siglo XI*. Barcelona: Sobs. De López Robert, 1943.

Ferre, Lola. "Epithymum for Melancholy: Two Prescriptions in a Treatise Attributed to Isaac al-Israeli." In *A Key to Locked Doors: Festschrift for Gerrit Bos*, edited by Fabian Käs, Jessica Kley, and F. Hedderich, 411–31. Leiden: Brill, 2024.

——. "Isaac Israeli's 'The Definition of Fever and its Essence' in its Hebrew Translations." *Transactions of the American Philosophical Society*, n.s., vol. 111, no. 5 (2023): 1–256.

——. *Práctica de Johannes de Parma: Un tratado farmacológico en sus versiones hebreas y catalana*. Granada: Universidad de Granada, 2002.

——. "La terminología médica en las versiones hebreas de textos latinos." *Miscelánea de estudios árabes y hebraicos* (MEAH), Hebr. section, 40 (1991): 87–107.

——. "Las traducciones hebreas de la obra médica de Bernard de Gordon." *Miscelánea de estudios árabes y hebraicos* (MEAH), Hebr. section, 49 (2000): 191–205.

Ferre, Lola, and Michael McVaugh. *The Tabula Antidotarii of Armengaud Blaise and its Hebrew Translation*. Philadelphia: American Philosophical Society, 2000.

Font Estrela, Jordi. "Las sátiras misóginas de Maimón Gallipapa: 'El Voto de la Viuda' y 'Querellas de una Mujer.'" *Miscelánea de estudios árabes y hebraicos* (MEAH), Hebrew section, 44 (1995): 149–70.

Franklin-Lyons, Adam, and Marie Kelleher. "Framing Mediterranean Famine: Food Crises in Fourteenth-Century Barcelona." *Speculum* 97, no. 1 (2022): 40–76.

Freudenthal, Gad, and Mauro Zonta. "Avicenna among Medieval Jews: The Reception of Avicenna's Philosophical, Scientific, and Medical Writings in Jewish Cultures East and West." *Arabic Sciences and Philosophy* 22 (2012): 217–87.

Friedenwald, Harry. *The Physicians' Aphorisms: A Medieval Hebrew Satire*. Baltimore, 1918. Repr. from *Johns Hopkins Hospital Bulletin* 29, no. 325, March 1918.

Galipapa, Maimon. "Physicians' Aphorisms" [in Hebrew]. In vol. 2 of Hayyim Schirmann, *HaShirah ha'Ivrit biSefarad uveProvanz*, 548–55. 4 vols. Jerusalem: Mossad Bialik and Dvir, 1956–1960.

García Ballester, Luis. "La recepción del Colliget de Averroes en Montpellier y su influencia en las polémicas sobre la naturaleza de la fiebre." In vol. 2 of *Homenaje al Profesor Dario Cabanelas Rodriguez*, edited by Luis García Ballester, 317–32. 2 vols. Granada: Universidad de Granada, 1987.

——. "Changes in the *Regimina Sanitatis*: The Role of Jewish Physicians." In *Health, Disease, and Healing in Medieval Culture*, edited by Sheila Campbell, Bert Hall, and David Klausner, 119–31. New York: Palgrave-MacMillan, 1992.

García Ballester, Luis, Lola Ferre, and Eduard Feliu. "Jewish Appreciation of Fourteenth-Century Scholastic Medicine." In *Renaissance Medical Learning: Evolution of a Tradition*, in *Osiris* 2nd ser., 6 (1990): 85–117.

Gil-Sotres, Pedro. "Derivation and Revulsion: The Theory and Practice of Medieval Phlebotomy." In *Practical Medicine from Salerno to the Black Death*, edited by Luis García Ballester, Jon Arrizabalaga, and Roger French, 110–55. Cambridge: Cambridge University Press, 1994.

——. "Sangre y patología en la medicina bajomedieval: El substrato material de la flebotomía." *Asclepio* 38 (1986): 73–104.

Green, Monica H. "The Four Black Deaths." *American Historical Review* 125, no. 5 (2020): 1600–1631.

——. "A New Definition of the Black Death: Genetic Findings and Historical Interpretations." *Medio aevo* 11, no. 2 (2022): 139–55.

——. "Out of the East (or North or South): A Response to Philip Slavin," *Past & Present* 256, no. 1 (2022): 283–323.

——. "Putting Africa on the Black Death Map: Narratives from Genetics and History." *Afriques* 9 (2018), https://doi.org/10.4000/afriques.2125.

Green, Monica H., and Andre Filipe Oliveira da Sliva. "Shifting Paradigms in Black Death Chronologies." *Hypotheses* (May 23, 2023), https://urbrel.hypotheses.org/5550.

Gross, Henri. *Gallia Judaica*. Paris: Cerf, 1897.

Guilleré, Christian. "La Peste noire à Girone." *Annals de l'Institut d'estudis gironins* 7 (1984): 87–161.

Gutwirth, Eleazar. "En Maymon Galipapa: Texto y contexto de un intelectual ilerdense (s. XIV)." In *Actes Ir. Colloqui d'Història dels Jueus a la Corona d'Aragó*, 339–48. Lleida: Institut d'Estudis Ilerdencs, 1991.

Gyug, Richard. "The Effects and Extent of the Black Death of 1348: New Evidence for Clerical Mortality in Barcelona." *Mediaeval Studies* 45, no. 1 (1983): 385–96.

Harris, Nichola. "The Protection of Innocents: Red Coral as a Lapidary Cure for the 'Children's Disease' and Conditions Related to Childbirth in Medieval and Early Modern England." In *Death and Disease in the Medieval and Early Modern World: Perspectives from Across the Mediterranean and Beyond*, edited by Lori Jones and Nükhet Varlık, 265–92. Woodbridge: York Medieval/Boydell, 2022.

Hymes, Robert, and Monica H. Green. *New Evidence for the Dating and Impact of the Black Death in Asia*, edited by Carol Symes. *The Medieval Globe*. Leeds: Arc Humanities, 2022.

Jacquart, Danielle. "Les avatars de la phrénitis chez Avicenne et Rhazès." In *La science médicale occidentale entre deux renaissances (XIIe s.–XVe s.)*, edited by Danielle Jacquart, 181–92, Essay IX. Hampshire: Aldershot Variorum, 1997.

Jones, Lori. "Bubo Men? Repurposing Medieval Anatomic Illustrations for Plague Therapy in the Fifteenth and Sixteenth Centuries." In *Death and Disease in the Medieval and Early Modern World: Perspectives from Across the Mediterranean and Beyond*, edited by Lori Jones and Nükhet Varlik, 221–46. Woodbridge: York Medieval/Boydell, 2022.

——. *Patterns of Plague: Changing Ideas about Plague in England and France*. Montreal: McGill/Queen's University Press, 2022.

Jordan, William C. "Administering Expulsion in 1306." *Jewish Studies Quarterly* 15, no. 3 (2008): 241–50.

——. *The French Monarchy and the Jews*. Philadelphia: University of Pennsylvania Press, 1989.

——. *The Great Famine: Northern Europe in the Early Fourteenth Century*. Princeton: Princeton University Press, 1996.

Kacki, Sacha, and Dominique Castex. "La sépulture multiple de la basilique des Saints Martyrs Just et Pastor: Bio-archéologie des restes humaines." *Quarhis: Quaderns d'arqueologia i història de la ciutat de Barcelona* 2, no. 10 (2014): 180–99.

Kahl, Oliver, ed. and transl. *Sābūr ibn Sahl: The Small Dispensatory*. Leiden: Brill, 2003.

Kelleher, Marie. *The Hungry City: A Year in the Life of Medieval Barcelona*. Ithaca: Cornell University Press, 2025.

Keller, Marcel, Meriam Guellil, Philip Slavin, et al. "A Refined Chronology of the Second Plague Pandemic in Western Eurasia." preprint *bioRxv* (July 19, 2023), https://doi.org/10.1101/2023.07.18.549544.

Lafuente Gómez, Mario. "La conquista y colonización de Cerdeña por la Corona de Aragón: Historiografías nacionales, investigaciones recientes y renovación interpretativa." *Rivista dell' Istituto di storia dell' Europa mediterranea*, n.s., vol. 6 (June 2020): 105–45.

Langermann, Y. Tzvi. "Maimonides on the Synochous Fever." *Israel Oriental Studies* 13 (1993): 175–98.

Lardos, Andreas, Kristina Patmore, Robert Allkin, et al. "A Systematic Methodology to Assess the Identity of Plants in Historical Texts: A Case Study Based on the Byzantine Pharmacy Text John the Physician's *Therapeutics*." *Journal of Ethnopharmacology* 322 (2024): 1–18.

Lev, Efraim, and Zohar Amar. "Reconstruction of the Inventory of *Materia medica* Used by Members of the Jewish Community in Medieval Cairo." *Journal of Ethnopharmacology* 108 (2006): 428–44.

Maltas i Montoro, Joan. *Caresties, fams i epidemies a Catalunya: De la conquesta de Sicilia a la Pesta Negra*. Lleida: Pagès, 2022.

Marganne, Marie-Hélène. "Sur l'origine Hippocratique des concepts de révulsion et de dérivation." *L'Antiquité classique* 49 (1980): 115–30.
McVaugh, Michael. "Bedside Manners in the Middle Ages." *Bulletin of the History of Medicine* 71, no. 2 (1997): 201–23.
——. "The 'humidium radicale' in Thirteenth-century Medicine." *Traditio* 30 (1974): 259–83.
——. *Medicine before the Plague: Practitioners and their Patients in the Crown of Aragon*, 1285–1345. Cambridge: Cambridge University Press, 2002.
——. "El món mèdic de Castelló d'Empúries a principis del segle XIV." *Mot so razo* 10–11 (2012):7–16.
McVaugh, Michael, Gerrit Bos, and Joseph Shatzmiller. *The Regimen sanitatus of "Avenzoar": Stages in the Production of a Medieval Translation*. Leiden: Brill, 2019.
Meyerhof, Max. "Esquisse d'histoire de la pharmacologie et botanique chez les musulmans d'Espagne." *Al-Andalus* 3, no. 1 (1935): 1–41.
Miret y Sans, Joaquín. "Les médecins juifs de Pierre, roi d'Aragon." *Revue des études juives* 57, no. 114 (1909): 268–78.
Muntané i Santiveri, Josep Xavier. "Aproximació a les causes de l'avalot de Tàrrega de 1348." *Tamid: Revista catalana annual d'estudis hebraics* 8 (2012): 105–29.
——. "Itinerari pels documents relatius a l'assalt del call de Tàrrega de l'any 1348." *Urtx* 23 (2009): 158–79.
Nash, Linda. "Beyond Virgin Soil Epidemics." In *Oxford Handbook of Environmental History*, edited by Andrew C. Isenberg, 76–102. Oxford: Oxford University Press, 2014.
Nicoud, Marilyn. "À l'épreuve de la peste: Médecins et savoirs médicaux face à la pandémie (XIV–XVe s.)." *Annales HSS* 78, no. 3 (2023): 505–41.
Oliveira da Silva, Andre. "Chronologies, Routes and Conditions for the Spread of Plague in Portugal During the Black Death." *Anais de história de Além-Mar* 22 (2021): 59–84.
Peña Muñoz, Carmen, and F. Girón Irueste. "The Identification of Fevers According to al-Isra'īli, Avenzoar, and Bernard Gordon." *Cronos* 8 (2005): 95–120.
Phillips, William D. "Peste Negra: The Fourteenth-Century Plague Epidemics in Iberia." In *On the Social Origins of Medieval Institutions*, edited by Donald Kagay and T. M. Vann, 47–62. Leiden: Brill, 1998.
Pinkhof, H. *Abraham Kashlari over Pestachtige Koortsen. Hebreeuwsch met Nederlandsche Vertaling. Naar het te Leidenvoorhanden handschrift, benevens een bericht over vier andere 14e eeuwsche Hebreeuwsche handschriften, handelende overde pest*. Amsterdam, 1891.
Pormann, Peter, and Emilie Savage-Smith, eds. *Medieval Islamic Medicine*. Washington, DC: Georgetown University Press, 2007.
Rasmussen, Simon, Morten Erik Allentoft, Kasper Nielsen, et al. "Early Divergent Strains of *Yersinia Pestis* in Eurasia 5000 Years Ago." *Cell* 153 (2015): 571–82.
Reixach-Sala, Albert. "Fighting the Plague in the Crown of Aragon (Mid-Fourteenth to Early Sixteenth Century)." *Journal of Medieval Iberian Studies*, Jan. 13, 2025, https://doi.org/10.1080/17546559.2024.2422034.
Renan, Ernst. *Écrivains juifs français du XIVe s*. Paris: Imprimerie nationale, 1893.
Richler, Benjamin. "Manuscripts of Avicenna's Kanon in Hebrew Translation: A Revised and Up-to-date List," *Korot* 8, nos. 3–4 (1982): 145*–68* (asterisk indicates English section), 137–43 in Hebrew.

Romeu Ferré, Pilar. *Tratado sobre la peste: Edición critica del manuscrito 2726 del Jewish Theological Seminary of America (siglo XV)*. Barcelona: Tirocinio, 2024.

Rosner, Fred. *Moses Maimonides' Glossary of Drug Names*. Philadelphia: American Philosophical Society, 1979.

Savage-Smith, Emilie. "Were the Four Humours Fundamental to Medieval Islamic Medical Practice?" In *The Body in Balance: Humoral Theory in Practice*, edited by Peregrine Horden and Elisabeth Hsu, 89–106. New York: Bergahn, 2013.

Schirmann, Hayyim (Jefim). *HaShirah ha'Ivrit biSefarad uveProvanz*. 4 vols. Jerusalem: Mossad Bialik and Dvir, 1956–1960.

Secord, James A. "Knowledge in Transit." *Isis* 95, no. 4 (2004): 654–72.

Shatzmiller, Joseph. "Apprenticeship or Academic Education: The Making of Jewish Doctors." In *Schüler und Meister*, edited by Andreas Speer and Thomas Jeschke, 503–10. Berlin: De Gruyter, 2016.

Slavin, Philip. "Out of the West: Formation of a Permanent Plague Reservoir in South-Central Germany (1349–1356) and Its Implications." *Past & Present* 252, no. 1 (2021): 3–51.

Smail, Daniel Lord. "A Life in the Black Death: The Inventory of Alayseta Paula (Marseille 1348)." *Middle Ages for Educators*, April 1, 2020. https://middleagesforeducators.princeton.edu/life-black-death-inventory-alayseta-paula-marseille-1348, accessed Dec. 1, 2025.

Spyrou, Maria, Lyazzat Musralina, Guido A. Gnecchi Ruscone, et al. "The Source of the Black Death in Fourteenth-Century Central Eurasia." *Nature* 606 (2022): 718–24.

Stearns, Justin. *Infectious Ideas: Contagion in Premodern Islamic and Christian Thought in the Western Mediterranean*. Baltimore: Johns Hopkins University Press, 2011.

Van Arsdall, Anne. *Medieval Herbal Remedies: The "Old English Herbarium" and Early Medieval Medicine*. 2nd ed. Abingdon: Routledge, 2023.

Varlik, Nükhet. "Four Colours of Disease and Death in the Early Modern Ottoman Cultural Imagination." In *Death and Disease in the Medieval and Early Modern World: Perspectives from Across the Mediterranean and Beyond*, edited by Lori Jones and Nükhet Varlik, 123–48. Woodbridge: York Medieval/Boydell, 2022.

——. *Plague and Empire in the Early Modern Mediterranean World: The Ottoman Experience 1347–1600*. Cambridge: Cambridge University Press, 2015.

Voigts, Linda, and Michael McVaugh. "A Latin Technical Phlebotomy and its Middle English Translation." *Transactions of the American Philosophical Society* 74, no. 2 (1984): 1–69.

Waal, Alex de. "Hunger in Global War Economies: Understanding the Decline and Return of Famines." *Disasters* 49 no. 1 (2024): e12661, https://doi.org/10.1111/disa.12661.

——. *Mass Starvation: The History and Future of Famine*. New York: Wiley, 2017.

——. "Memory and the Social Meanings of Famine." *Third World Quarterly* 45, no. 2 (2024): 439–43.

Wallis, Faith. "Signs and Senses: Diagnosis and Prognosis in Early Medieval Pulse and Urine Texts." *Social History of Medicine* 13, no. 2 (2000): 265–78.

Weiss, Daniel. "Bronze Age Plague," *Archaeology* Jan/Feb 2019. https://archaeology.org/issues/january-february-2019/collection/russia-samara-bronze-age-plague/top-10-discoveries-of-2018/, accessed Dec. 1, 2025.